Combating
Allergy Naturally

I0125765

Dr. A K Sethi

V&SPUBLISHERS

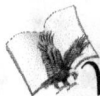

Published by:

V&S PUBLISHERS

F-2/16, Ansari road, Daryaganj, New Delhi-110002
☎ 23240026, 23240027 • *Fax:* 011-23240028
Email: info@vspublishers.com • *Website:* www.vspublishers.com

Branch: Hyderabad
5-1-707/1, Brij Bhawan (Beside Central Bank of India Lane)
Bank Street, Koti Hyderabad - 500 095
☎ 040-24737290
E-mail: vspublishershyd@gmail.com

Distributors:

► **Pustak Mahal®**, Delhi
J-3/16, Daryaganj, New Delhi-110002
☎ 23276539, 23272783, 23272784 • *Fax:* 011-23260518
E-mail: sales@pustakmahal.com • *Website:* www.pustakmahal.com
Bengaluru: ☎ 080-22234025 • *Telefax:* 080-22240209
Patna: ☎ 0612-3294193 • *Telefax:* 0612-2302719

► **PM Publications**
• 10-B, Netaji Subhash Marg, Daryaganj, New Delhi-110002
☎ 23268292, 23268293, 23279900 • *Fax:* 011-23280567
E-mail: pmpublications@gmail.com
• 6686, Khari Baoli, Delhi-110006
☎ 23944314, 23911979

► **Unicorn Books**
Mumbai:
23-25, Zaoba Wadi (Opp. VIP Showroom), Thakurdwar, Mumbai-400002
☎ 022-22010941 • *Telefax:* 022-22053387

© **Copyright:** V&S PUBLISHERS
ISBN 978-93-813846-1-9
Edition: 2011

Printed at : Parma Offsetters, Okhla, New Delhi

Preface

Allergy is the bane of our modern civilisation and has assumed epidemic proportions in all parts of the world. It poses one of the greatest health challenges of the 21st century, because no curative treatment has been found so far. Moreover, with scientific advancement, the menace of environmental pollution has also contributed towards the problem of Allergy.

Allergies are of several types. Some individuals are allergic to dust and changes in temperature; others are adversely affected by certain food substances or medicines. A few people suffer from skin allergy and a handful develop allergic symptoms due to insects and even their pet animals.

Since Allopathic treatment has failed to find a cure for the curse of Allergy, it is worthwhile trying other alternative forms of treatment like Ayurveda, Yoga, Homeopathy, Naturopathy, Magnetotherapy, Colour Therapy, Acupressure, Music Therapy, Vastu Shastra and Feng Shui.

I have ventured to write this book in order to educate the layman about the different aspects of Allergy and hope the readers will find it useful and enjoyable to read. For any queries and clarification, readers are free to contact me on telephone no. **(011) 27044226 or 9811506972** or mail to *Sethi62in@yahoo.com.*

Acknowledgement

At the outset, I must thank my publishers **M/s Pustak Mahal** for giving me the opportunity to write this book for the layman on an ailment which is widely prevalent around the globe, but there is no known cure for it.

I am grateful to the patients who came to our clinic for treatment of Allergy and benefitted from the alternative forms of treatment. I am indebted to the following experts in the Alternative therapies, i.e. Shri RL Jaggi - Colour Therapy, Swami Ananta Bharati - Yoga, Shri NS Dabas - Vastu Shastra and Magnetotherapy, Dr Ruma Banerjee - Naturopathy and Physiotherapy, Dr RK Kumar - Homeopathy.

My special thanks to Shri SK Gaba for providing me the latest material on the modern as well as alternative therapies of Allergy. Mrs Kiran Arora has done the tedious task of computer typing, scanning and compiling the book.

My wife Dr. Sunanda Sethi, an Ayurvedacharya and a Reiki Grandmaster, has been a continuous source of inspiration for me. I thank my children Rupal and Mitali, without whose cooperation this book would not have been completed.

–Dr A K Sethi

Contents

1

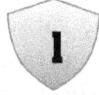

What is Allergy

When we mention the word "Allergy", majority of people correlate it with **"Aachoo"** – sneezing, running nose, watering of eyes, cough, etc. Some people think of allergy to medicines like Penicillin, Sulfa drugs, etc. and others connect it to food substances like milk, meat, cheese, etc.

Unfortunately, allergy has become the bane of modern civilisation and we find ourselves allergic to several substances like pets, insects, perfumes, wheat, food preservatives, latex (gloves), plants, metals like arsenic, etc. Allergy is also a complicated and enigmatic subject for doctors and scientists, since neither the causative mechanism is clear, nor the treatment is satisfactory.

In order to understand what allergy is all about, we must first understand its basic mechanism. Allergy is closely related to our Immune System – the system which protects us from sickness and diseases. Our body is so designed that whenever a foreign invader (bacteria, virus, chemical, heat, cold, wind, water, etc.) or inner enemy (tumour, aged cells, etc.) attacks our body, the immune system gets activated to protect us from this invader.

The innate (inborn) immune system consists of barriers such as skin and mucous membranes, enzymes and white blood cells (WBC) called neutrophils in its armamentarium. If the innate immune system is unsuccessful, the adaptive immune system takes over.

This system consists of cells such as lymphocytes and monocytes and their products such as antibodies, cytokines and antigen-specific cytotoxic (killer) cells. This system does not damage the body tissues, but destroys the abnormal material (invader). It also remembers the encounters with specific invaders such that subsequent encounters by the host with the same agents activate the immune response more quickly and vigorously, preventing recurrence of the disease caused by the invader.

In contrast to the adaptive immune system, in certain individuals there is an over-reactive immune system, i.e. there is an abnormal reaction to the ordinarily harmless substances (invaders). This disorder is called an **Allergy** or **Hypersensitivity**.

What Happens During an Allergic Reaction

When a person with a hypersensitive or hyper-alert immune system is exposed to an invader (an allergen), a series of events take place:-

1. The WBC of the body start to produce a specific type of antibodies called Immunoglobulin E (IgE) to fight the allergen.

2. These antibodies attach to another types of cells called mast cells, which are found in the airways and in the digestive system where the allergens enter the body.

3. The mast cells release a variety of chemicals like histamine, serotonin, etc. which produce localised effects like sneezing, running nose, watery eyes, itching, diarrhoea, vomiting, etc. or generalised effects like breathing difficulty, low blood pressure, swelling of body, weakness, loss of consciousness, shock or even death.

There are two major differences between the normal immune reaction and allergic reaction:-

1. In a normal individual there is an antigen-antibody reaction, which protects the individual (host) while in a person with allergy, the reaction of allergen with

tissue-bound antibody (IgE) can lead to several unpleasant symptoms to the body and causation of disease.

2. In an allergic person, the body does not produce antibodies (IgE) unless he has been sufficiently exposed to the allergen earlier and for a prolonged period. Hence in cases of Food Allergy, the person who has been eating the (allergic) food substance regularly is more prone to develop a reaction than to a new substance recently added to his diet.

There is another type of allergic reaction seen in allergic individuals, which is known as **Delayed Hypersensitivity Reaction** or **Cellular Allergy**. In this case, the body, instead of producing IgE antibodies, has overreactive lymphocytes produced by thymus gland. When exposed to certain allergic substances which come into direct contact with the skin, this type of allergic reaction is observed. The lymphocytes while reacting to get rid of the foreign material or toxin give rise to certain skin changes causing a disease called **Contact Dermatitis**.This type of allergic reaction is also seen when the body rejects the organs transplanted in the body.

●●

2

Types of Allergies

As written earlier, allergy is of different types depending on the mechanism of action and the offending agent (allergen). For a layman it will be easier to comprehend if allergy is classified based on the causative agent. Thus the types of allergy may be classified as given below:-

❑ Dust Allergy

❑ Food Allergy

❑ Drug Allergy

❑ Insect Allergy

❑ Skin Allergy

❑ Allergy due to other substances

Dust Allergy

Dust allergy refers to allergic symptoms caused by inhaling (breathing in) certain microscopic particles found in the environment surrounding us. These allergens (also called aeroallergens) may be found either at home, in our place of work or while travelling from one place to another. The common aeroallergens are as follows:

❑ Dust, smoke, fumes and gases emitted by polluting vehicles, industries and factories are most common aeroallergens in India.

10

- Climatic conditions like high humidity, sudden changes in temperature, especially from warm to cold and smog formation are also important factors causing allergic symptoms.
- Active and passive smoking is equally responsible for causing allergy and other symptoms of the respiratory system.
- Pollen grains of different plants suspended in air especially on windy and rainy days.
- Fungi and moulds found in damp and moist areas also cause allergic diseases.
- Dust mite found at home that collect in the mattresses, furniture, carpets and rugs, bedding draperies, clothes and floor, which are inhaled while dusting or cleaning the house.
- Inhalation of insect parts and droppings of cockroaches, flies, moths, butterflies, rats, mice, bed bugs, mosquitoes, houseflies, etc.
- Animal allergen in the form of epithelial scales (dander), hair or feathers of animals like dogs, cats, cattle, horse, sheep, goat, duck, etc.
- Occupational allergens like silica, asbestos, lead, nickel, coal, cotton, wool, fibres, paints, varnishes, resins, grain flour, formaldehyde, insecticides, pesticides, dyes, drugs, spices, printing ink, etc.

Food Allergy

Foods are mainly composed of proteins, carbohydrates and lipids. Usually, the major food allergens are the glycoproteins found in the food.

- About 2-3% of infants suffer from **cow's milk allergy**, which is the most common food allergy of childhood. This seems logical since cow's milk formula is usually the first foreign substance a baby consumes, and also the digestive and immune systems of the infant are not fully developed. Most children outgrow milk allergies by the age of four and food allergies that develop after this age are usually permanent. The major allergens in milk are the caseins and the whey protein – beta lactoglobulin. The milk from goats and sheep has almost similar proteins as cow's milk and cannot be used as the latter's substitute.

❏ Allergy to **eggs** is usually observed in young children and like cow's milk allergy, fades with time. The main allergens are the egg-white proteins, ovomucoid, ovalbumin and ovotransferrin. The eggs of other poultry such as ducks are similar to that of hens and also cause allergy.

❏ **Seafood** allergy is more common in adults than children and is more prevalent in countries with a high consumption of fish and shellfish. The major allergens in fish are flesh-proteins called parvalbumins, which are similar in all kinds of fish. Cooking does not destroy the allergens in fish and shellfish and some individuals may be allergic to the cooked and not raw fish.

❏ Certain **fruits** and **vegetables** are also capable of causing allergic reactions, though very mild and often limited to the mouth (oral-allergy syndrome). The commonly allergic fruits and vegetables are apples, bananas, tomatoes, soyabean, peas, and beans. Many of these allergens are destroyed by cooking and are thus safe in allergic individuals.

❏ **Peanuts** are one of the most allergenic food and frequently cause very severe reactions, including death. This allergy is established in childhood and is usually maintained throughout life. Traces of peanuts found in processed oils or in utensils used for serving foods, can be enough in some individuals to cause an allergic reaction.

- **Tree nuts** such as walnuts, almonds, cashewnuts, hazelnuts and pistachios can cause very severe allergic symptoms, which can occasionally be fatal. Roasting or cooking cannot destroy the allergens.

- Certain **cereals** like wheat, rice, barley, rye, oats and maize are also associated with allergy. The more we eat these cereals the more likely we are to suffer an allergy. Seed storage proteins such as wheat gluten and other proteins present in grain to protect it from bacteria and fungi have been found to be major allergens.

- **Food additives** and **preservatives** like sulfites, tartrazine, monosodium glutamate are also responsible for causing food allergy.

Drug Allergy

Almost everyone in his lifetime has undergone certain unpleasant effects due to medicines. Some may develop drowsiness, others develop stomach disorders like diarrhoea or constipation or hyperacidity and a few develop headache, giddiness, etc. These are usually the **known** side-effects due to overdose or drug-interactions. Drug allergy usually refers to serious adverse effects in a person, which **may not have occurred** while taking the same medicine earlier. The mechanism of these effects are due to production of Immunoglobulin E as in the case of other allergies. Usually people with drug allergies have a family history of allergies and may be also suffering from **dust allergy** or **food allergy.**

The medicines to which people usually develop drug allergy are as follows:–

1. Penicillin group and Cephalosporins

2. Insulin

3. Vaccines like DPT, Influenza (HIB), Tetanus, MMR, Chickenpox

4. Sulfonamides (Sulfa drugs)

5. Intravenous contrast, dyes used in tests like CT Scan, MRI, IVP, etc.
6. Aspirin and other painkillers
7. Local and general anaesthesia

Insect Allergy

Usually insect bites and stings cause mild and temporary pain and swelling at the site of the bites. In sensitised individuals, allergic reactions may result in more severe local reactions as well as generalised symptoms ranging from mild to fatal responses.

The insects which usually cause allergic symptoms are as follows:–

- ❑ Bees – honey bees, bumble bees
- ❑ Wasps, hornets, yellowjackets
- ❑ Fire ants
- ❑ Mosquitoes

The risk of insect bites increases in summer and rainy weather and can occur with outdoor exposure. Incidence is more in unsanitary areas, forests and grassy areas and near the water bodies. Loose fitting clothes may entrap insects. Insects are attracted to bright colours and floral patterns and to perfumes, lotions, scented soaps and hair preparations.

Skin Allergy

Several soaps, detergents, perfumes, cosmetics, dyes and items of daily use produce allergic reactions at the site of contact. This is referred to as skin allergy. The allergic effects are more common in thinner sites like eyelids, earlobes and genital sites, and less in palms of hands and soles of feet.

The following are the allergens and the sources where they are found:-

Substance	Source
Plants	Poison ivy, poison oak, chrysanthemum, tulips, rosewood pines.
Nickel	Jewellery, watches, jean studs, bra clips.
Rubber / Latex	Gloves, condoms, clothing, shoes, tyres.
Colophony	Sticking plaster, adhesives, sealants, collodion.
Epoxy resins	Adhesives, paints, surface coatings.
Wool alcohol (Lanolin)	Cosmetics, creams, ointments, lotions, soaps.
Paraphenylenediamine	Hair dye, shampoo, conditioners.
Balsam of Peru	Perfumes, citrus fruits
Neomycin	Ointment, cream, eye drops, lotions.
Furazoline	Furacin ointment.
Potassium dichromate	Cement, industrial chemicals.
Thiomerasol	Preservatives in cosmetics, nose drops and ear drops.

Allergy Due to Other Substances

Solar Allergy

Many people are allergic to sunlight and develop skin disease (dermatitis) within minutes of exposure to sunlight. The ultraviolet rays of the sun act as the trigger for allergic changes on the skin. Sometimes, sunscreening agents used in cosmetics such as moisturisers, lip and hair preparations and foundation make-up, accelerate solar allergy.

Allergy Towards Pets

Many people with a history of **dust** allergy or **food** allergy, who keep pets at home, have been observed to have allergic symptoms due to the pets. Dogs and cats are such faithful and lovable animals that millions of people keep them as pets at home. Majority of people play with them or bathe them or even make them stay in their bedroom, without facing any problems. But certain individuals immediately start sneezing and coughing when they enter the room where the animals are located. Such people are known to suffer from pet allergy. The allergens in dogs are the dead skin flakes or epithelial scales and in the cat, the sebum from the sebaceous glands near the base of the tail. Hair or feathers from cattle, horse, sheep, goat, duck and other birds also have an allergic effect. Urine, saliva and bacteria of these animals as well as rats and mice can also cause allergy.

••

3

Effects of Allergy on the Body

Dust Allergy

Dust allergy refers to allergic symptoms caused by airborne particles in our environment like pollen grains, house dust, cockroach and insect parts, fungi and moulds, indoor and outdoor smoke, fumes and other pollutants, climatic changes and viruses and bacteria.

These airborne particles can affect different parts of the body, i.e. nose, sinuses, ears, lungs and eyes.

Nasal Allergy or Allergic Rhinitis: People complain of sneezing, itching of the nose, nasal blockage with intermittent watering of the nose. Some people also develop increased watering of the eyes, itching and redness of the eyes. A few people develop headache, bodyache, malaise, fatigue and irritability. With the passage of time, the nasal secretions become dry and enter the throat to cause sore throat with development of dry cough. Recent research suggests that many children with nasal allergy also have poor school performance and absenteeism from school.

Allergy of the Sinuses or Allergic Sinusitis: Paranasal sinuses are empty spaces around the nose, which are usually filled up with air. There is severe headache in the frontal region and swelling around the nose, especially in the morning. This headache becomes less as the day advances. There is watering of nose with secretions, which may be yellow or green in colour. There may be sneezing or itching in the nose and sore throat in some. Some people may complain of loss of taste or smell. If the condition is not treated, fever may occur due to super-added bacterial infection.

Allergic Symptoms of the Ear and Throat: Dust allergy can also affect the Eustachian tube (ear) and throat. Children with allergy of the ears complain of acute earache on one side, usually occurring early in the morning. These children are usually irritable, may have fever and occasionally nausea, vomiting and diarrhoea.

In the case of allergy of the throat, there is a sticky sensation or pain in the throat, especially while swallowing solids. There may be dry cough and sometimes fever and a sensation of vomiting.

Allergic Symptoms of the Eye: Itching is the hallmark of allergy of the eye that can last from a few hours to many days. It may be mild or severe with clear, watery discharge from the eye. Most environmental allergen exposures are associated with symptoms affecting both eyes. Sometimes sharp and piercing pain of the eyes and swelling of eyelids may also occur.

Allergic Asthma: Dust allergy usually affects the lungs and the condition is known as allergic asthma. Those who suffer from this condition complain of recurrent episodes of wheezing – high-pitched musical or whistling sounds heard during exhalation. Such individuals have a feeling of tightness around the chest and coughing, particularly at night or in the early morning. They have difficulty in breathing even when they are immobile. The condition may deteriorate and nebuliser may be required in many cases. Asthma, being a genetic disease, is associated with other types of allergy, especially skin allergy. Usually one or more parents may be suffering from some type of allergy. This disease is more common and intense during childhood and sometimes becomes latent or disappears during adulthood. Changes in weather conditions, especially a humid or rainy weather precipitates allergic asthma in most sensitive individuals.

Food Allergy

Food allergy refers to the outcome of immune response following food intake, whereas **food intolerance** refers to toxic contaminants in food or stale, uncooked or undigested food, lack of digestive enzymes or due to psychological reasons.

Reaction to foods is usually rapid, appearing within an hour (or sometimes even in seconds) of consumption, though it may appear after up to four hours in some cases. The reaction to food may appear in the oral region, in the digestive system, respiratory system, eyes, skin or all over the body. The usual symptoms of food allergy are as follows:-

❑ In the oral region, itching and swelling of the lips, tongue, palate and throat may be observed. The symptoms are often associated with intake of various fruits and vegetables. Patients with nasal allergy due to ragweed may develop symptoms after intake of melons and bananas. Similarly, patients sensitive to birch pollen may develop oral symptoms due to intake of raw potatoes, carrots, celery, apples and hazelnuts. The symptoms generally resolve rapidly.

❑ Symptoms in the digestive system develop within minutes to two hours of eating the offending food. The symptoms are nausea, vomiting, abdominal cramps, bloating and diarrhoea.

❑ In the respiratory system, people with food allergy experience itching in the nose, sneezing, a runny nose and wheezing, breathlessness, voice changes and coughing. Inhalation of a food allergen while cooking or during food processing can cause severe asthmatic symptoms.

❑ Some people develop itching, watering and redness of the eyes.

❑ The skin is a frequent target organ of food allergy. The most common skin manifestation of food allergy are skin rashes, such as nettle rash (also called urticaria or hives) appearing within minutes of consumption of food allergen. These skin reactions disappear within a few days. Some people develop long-lasting scaly patches, which have a relapsing course and are associated with asthma and nasal allergy.

❏ A few people with food allergy develop shock-like state with low-blood pressure, weak pulse, irregular heartbeat and sometimes death. People with peanut allergy have often had a fatal result.

Allergy to Medicines (Drug Allergy)

Allergy to medicines occurs mainly by two mechanisms – Immunoglobulin E-mediated reaction and cellular allergy (T-cell hypersensitivity). In the case of the former reaction, there has to be an adequate time of exposure to generate the immunoglobulins and in many cases the first exposure does not produce allergy. The signs and symptoms of drug allergy do not resemble known pharmacologic effects of the drug or the disease being treated. Penicillin allergy is the most common drug allergy seen today. Cellular allergy is seen mostly as skin allergy to poison oak, adhesive tape and several skin creams and ointments.

Insulin Allergy: Insulin is the most widely used human hormone used in the treatment of diabetes and is associated with allergic reactions due to its protein nature. Reaction to insulin at the site of injection occurs in about 5% to 10% of patients. There is pain, swelling and itching at the place of injection, which may progress to a larger swelling which persists for many days. In some people, rashes develop all over the body and there are adverse changes in the blood pressure, breathing pattern and digestive system.

Penicillin Allergy: Many people suffer from penicillin allergy and there have been fatal results with penicillin injections, especially those given intravenously. Skin test with penicillin injection is a must for all cases, **even those who have received this injection earlier without any**

reaction. Those who are allergic to penicillin injections are invariably allergic to oral penicillins like Ampicillin, Amoxicillin and the family of Cephalosporins like Cephalexin, Cefadroxil, etc. However, allergic reactions to these medicines are milder and not fatal.

Sulfa Allergy: Sulfa allergy is also common in many people though reactions are not always fatal.

Aspirin Allergy: Aspirin is second to penicillins as a cause of drug allergy. People with allergic asthma or nasal allergy have an increase in their symptoms when they take aspirin for fever, bodyache, headache, etc. (These symptoms occur after about two to three hours of intake of aspirin. Thus there may be increase in running nose, redness of eyes, cough, breathlessness and headache on taking aspirin. Rashes all over the body may develop in some cases. In others, there may be swelling all over the body with abdominal pain, low blood pressure and hoarseness of voice.

Allergy to Anaesthetic Agents

In people undergoing minor or major surgeries, local and general anaesthetic agents are used to reduce pain during surgery. Some individuals are allergic to these anaesthetic agents. The symptoms are sometimes manageable such as pain and swelling at the injection site, low blood pressure, increased heart rate, skin rashes, breathing difficulty, abdominal pain, and sometimes the results are fatal.

Allergy to Vaccines

Vaccines are used for prevention of different diseases. Many individuals are allergic to these vaccines due to different constituents of the vaccines.

❑ Due to the presence of egg protein in the vaccine some individuals are allergic to Yellow Fever and Influenza vaccines.

❑ Due to presence of mercury as a preservative, allergy to DPT (Diphtheria Pertussis Tetanus) and HIB (Haemophilus Influenza B) vaccines is observed.

- ❏ Due to presence of certain antibiotics, allergy to MMR (Measles Mumps Rubella), Chickenpox and OPV (Oral Polio Vaccine) are reported.
- ❏ Due to presence of gelatin, allergy to MMR and Chickenpox may be seen.
- ❏ Due to presence of infectious agent, Tetanus vaccine may prove to be allergic.

To administer any of the above vaccines, a test dose should be given to prevent allergic and untoward results due to the vaccines.

Allergy to Intravenous Contrast/Dyes

In some diseases, in order to get a clearer picture of the disease, certain dyes or contrast-media are injected into the blood. These contrast-media are used for getting CT Scan, MRI, IVP and other tests done. Sometimes allergic reactions in the form of disorder of kidney, lungs or heart, or even death may occur in about 5-8% of patients. So proper testing of these dyes should be done to avoid untoward reactions or other alternative tests can be done.

Insect Bite Allergy

There are several insects whose bites and stings cause localised and generalised allergic effects. Normally, there is itching, pain, burning, redness and mild swelling at the place where an insect bites. This reaction is caused by several chemically active components in the saliva or venom of the insect. This reaction usually subsides in a few hours and in people with sensitive skin, in a few days.

In allergic individuals, the swelling is larger and spreads throughout the limb. The surrounding lymph nodes in the armpit and thigh may also become swollen and painful.

Sometimes there is infection and pus formation at the place of bite, associated with fever. In serious cases, there is a feeling of tightness of throat, breathlessness, cough, giddiness, low blood pressure and unconsciousness. Children are less prone to develop serious allergic effects as compared to adults. Following several uneventful stings, serious reactions to insect stings develop subsequently.

In India, mosquito bite allergy is the commonest type of insect allergy but results are rarely fatal.

Skin Allergy

Skin allergy affects at least 15% of the general population at some time or the other during their lifetime and is the most frustrating type of allergy as far as treatment is concerned. Patient frequently go from one doctor to another in the hope of finding an extraordinary doctor who will be able to identify the cause, eliminate the culprit and exorcise them from this ailment.

Skin allergy is seen in three forms:-

❏ Atopic Dermatitis
❏ Contact Dermatitis
❏ Atopic Urticaria

Atopic Dermatitis is seen in early childhood, occuring before 5 years of age in about 90% of patients. This is characterised by large, red patches, which are very itchy and occur in the folds of arms, back of knees, cheeks, scalp, back of neck and trunk. This disease has a relapsing course – occuring several times, especially in summer and rainy weather. People who are of an anxious or hostile personality are more prone to this disease. This disease can also affect the eye leading to itching, burning and watering of the eyes with poor vision. This dermatitis is often associated with food allergens like milk, egg, peanut, soy, wheat, fish, and nuts like walnut, cashewnut, etc. House dust and animal dander act as air-borne allergens in many of these cases.

Contact Dermatitis refers to several signs of skin allergy induced by direct exposure to external substances. The common allergens responsible are plants like poison ivy, ragweed, tulips, rosewood, pine, metals, chemicals, dyes, resins, medicines and perfumes. The body's exposed areas,

23

especially the hands and face are the sites most frequently and at times exclusively involved with contact dermatitis. In the hand, the disease is more common between fingers and dorsal part of hand and less on the palms.

Atopic Dermatitis of the eyelids occurs more commonly due to cosmetics applied in other areas of the body, e.g., nails and scalp, than directly. Shampoos, conditioners, hair sprays, gel, eyelash curlers (nickel) and tissue papers containing fragrances, formaldehyde or benzylkonium chloride cause dermatitis of the eyelids. Face may be involved due to moisturisers, sunscreens, foundations, talcum powder, rubber sponges, masks, balloons, toys, etc.

The skin of the neck is vulnerable to irritant reactions from chemicals used in curling preparations, hair dyes, shampoos, conditioners and perfumes. Sensitivity to nail polish often presents as eczema of the neck rather than hand dermatitis. Nickel-sensitive individuals may react from wearing a necklace or from zippers. Deodorants can cause dermatitis of the axilla while certain clothes cause allergy in other surroundings areas. Shaving gels, after-shave lotions and hair-removing creams, and sometimes shaving creams, moisturisers and elastic socks can cause contact dermatitis of legs.

The anogenital area is also prone to develop contact dermatitis due to a variety of allergic agents. These include antibiotic creams, lotions, ointments, fragrances used in toilet paper, soaps, condoms, diaphragms and orally used laxatives, antibiotics and even spices.

Atopic Urticaria is usually referred to small or large patches/rashes which occur on different parts of the body due to allergic substances, e.g. swelling of the lips, or patches/rashes on the forehead due to allergic substances.

Solar Allergy

This is known in medical parlance as **Photo-contact Dermatitis**. This allergy is seen in individuals who have the inherent mechanism of absorbing the ultraviolet rays of the sun through the skin surface and underlying tissues. This type of allergy is seen in sun-exposed areas of the body like the face, front of the neck, back of the hands and forearms. These are very typically demarcated areas exposed to the sun where typical skin changes are seen.

Allergy Towards Pets

Most of the pet owners may have no health problems related to these pets. But some individuals, when they walk into the room where the cat or dog is located, suddenly start sneezing and have watering of the eyes and nose. They are said to suffer from pet allergy. The main cause of the allergic reaction is the presence of dead skin called dander and old skin scales suspended in the room where the pet is located. Usually the problem becomes worse during grooming, dusting, vacuuming or cleaning the animal's litter box. In addition, if the pet sleeps on the bed or pillows, the allergic reaction is worse at night or in the morning. In the case of cat, the allergen is found under the skin and near the base of the tail and is called Fel d1. This allergen is found in the dried sebaceous gland secretion and being small and light can be easily transferred into the clothing, carpet, and furniture or from person to person.

●●

4

Signs and Symptoms of Allergy

Allergy is a very complicated condition and is still not understood completely. The signs and symptoms are often related to the type of allergy and at times may be vague and hard to believe. Each type of allergy is explained with the help of case studies.

Dust Allergy

> *Whenever there were rains, Sania would start sneezing uncontrollably on waking up in the morning. Her eyes and nose would start watering incessantly and would become reddish and sore. By evening she would complain of itching in the throat and by next morning there would be severe cough and even fever. When Sania consulted a doctor, he informed her that she was suffering from Dust Allergy and this would usually be aggravated during humid weather conditions.*

Thus from the above case-study, the signs and symptoms of dust allergy are well evident. Besides the above symptoms, some people complain of itching in the eyes, nose and ears which are very significant for dust allergy. Headache, bodyache, malaise, fatigue and irritability is sometimes present. When dust allergy affects the lungs, it is known as **Allergic Asthma**. In this condition the common symptoms

26

are difficulty in breathing, wheezing or whistling sounds heard while breathing, coughing with sputum formation and a feeling of tightness in the chest. Some of these individuals may also have signs of skin allergy and may be allergic to aspirin.

Food Allergy

In the USA, food allergy occurs in 6-8% of children and 1-2% of adults. About 15% of the general population believe that they may be allergic to some food. Majority of food-allergic reactions present in the first year of life.

> *Mrs. Batra noticed that whenever they gave a treat of Cheese Pizza and Chocolate Ice-Cream to Rohan, he complained of stomach-ache and headache and was very irritable and tired for about 24-48 hours. When they consulted a gastroenterologist, he suggested that cheese and chocolate could be the culprits. Rohan was diagnosed as a case of food allergy.*

The most important aspect of food allergy is to remember that the signs and symptoms are not localised to the digestive system, but may occur in other parts of the body too. Some people with food allergy may develop itching and swelling around the lips and tongue after consuming **melons, bananas, carrots, celery, apples, hazelnuts** and **raw potatoes.** These symptoms may often be very mild and undetected and may resolve without any medicines. Others may develop nausea, vomiting, stomach-ache or cramps and diarrhoea within a few minutes to two hours after eating the allergic food items. Itching in the eyes, redness and watering may be seen in some. Some people have attacks of sneezing, running nose, coughing, hoarseness of voice, breathlessness and cough. Skin allergy is a very common effect of food allergy commonly seen with **fish, nuts** and **peanuts.** In very few individuals, food allergy may be fatal leading to weakness, low blood pressure and collapse.

Drug Allergy

Allergy to medicines varies according to the medicine given, the route by which given (oral or injections), dose and allergic susceptibility of the individual. Signs and symptoms of a few medicines are given below.

Allergy to **insulin** injection is often seen as a mild itching, swelling and pain at the site of injection which may subside within an hour of injection. In some, the allergy may be severe with itching all over the body and increase in the swelling, and pain persisting for more than two weeks.

Important clues of **latex allergy** are itching or swelling around the mouth after dental check-up or after blowing up balloons, local swelling or itching after vaginal or rectal examination or after use of condoms or itching of hands after coming into contact with any substance made of latex.

Individuals with allergy to **aspirin** usually develop running nose, sneezing, redness of eyes, wheezing and cough resembling sinusitis or asthma. Some individuals may develop skin problems, hoarse voice, abdominal pain and low blood pressure. Allergy to other medicines, especially **intravenous injections** and **anaesthetic** agents are often fatal in allergic individuals and hence a test dose should be given before administering the injection.

Insect Allergy

When Meenakshi Subramaniam delivered her first baby boy, everyone was overjoyed. The boy was so cute that everyone from the neighbourhood came to see him when he reached home. Suddenly, the next morning, Meenakshi saw that there were many red rashes all over the baby's face and body. She began to cry incessantly. Her husband immediately called the Child Specialist, Dr MK Sharma for his opinion. The doctor pacified them by saying that it was just insect allergy due to mosquito bites and they should use a mosquito net and repellant to protect the baby.

28

The normal reactions to insect bites and stings are itching, burning, pain, redness and mild swelling at the place of bite. In allergic individuals, the swelling continues to increase even after 6-8 hours and may involve a larger area with severe pain and redness. Some people have breathing problems, pain in the chest, cough, low blood pressure and may go into a state of shock. Children are less prone than adults to develop severe symptoms.

Skin Allergy

> *Rita was very happy when her husband presented her with a beautiful Titan watch for her birthday. She wore it to her office and everyone appreciated it. On returning home, she developed severe itching around her wrist. On removing the watch, she noticed that there was severe redness and swelling around her wrist. When she consulted a doctor, she came to know that it was a skin allergy due to the presence of nickel in the stainless steel strap.*

Skin allergy, as described earlier, is of two types – Atopic Dermatitis and Contact Dermatitis.

In **Atopic Dermatitis**, there is severe itching and redness and the disease is chronic and relapses from time to time. In children less than two years, the disease may be seen on the face and outer aspect of knees and elbows. In children above two years of age and in adults, the inner folds of arms and knees are involved. The other associated features are presence of allergy in other family members, seen in young age, influenced by environmental or emotional factors, itching associated with sweating and intolerance to wools and other irritants.

In **Contact Dermatitis**, the exposed areas of the body, especially the hands and face are most frequently and at times exclusively involved. The thinner sites like the eyelids, earlobes and genital skin are most vulnerable while thicker skin like the palms of hands and soles of feet are more resistant. Eyelids are a common target for contact dermatitis because of frequent exposures, increased susceptibility to irritants and allergens and easy accessibility to rubbing. Eyelids are more commonly involved due to cosmetics applied to other areas of the body like nails and scalp than to cosmetics directly applied to the eye area. Similarly, sensitivity to nail polish often affects the neck rather than hand.

Allergy towards Pets

> *Mr. Arora realised that whenever he came to the bedroom, he developed sneezing and running nose. This did not happen when he was in the other rooms. When he contacted Dr Chawla, their Family Physician, he realised that it was due to the addition of a new member in their family – Lucy, the cute Pomeranian puppy. Mr Arora was suffering from allergy due to the pet animal. When Lucy was given a separate kennel outside their house, this problem disappeared.*

Many people love to keep pets at home, but some of them may be suffering from allergy towards these animals. The symptoms associated with pet allergy usually include running nose, itching and watering of eyes, swollen eyelids, headache and sore-throat. For some people, an asthmatic attack may be triggered off when they are in close contact with their pet. They complain of tightness in the chest, shortness of breath, wheezing or whistling sounds in the chest and cough. This can sometimes be very serious and needs medical attention.

Solar Allergy

Some individual's skin is allergic to the ultraviolet rays of the sun. In such people, an eczema-like rash in seen in sun-exposed areas such as the forearms, back of hands, front of the neck and face. These rashes are well-demarcated and totally absent in those parts of the body which are always covered with clothing.

●●

5

Complications of Allergy

A llergy is also associated with several complications which may adversely affect the body of the patients. Children are more affected by complications due to their poor immunity and this also affects their school attendance and performance. Complications are also classified according to the type of allergy for better understanding of the subject.

Dust Allergy

If proper prevention and early treatment of dust allergy is not done, it may lead to several complications. There are certain empty spaces surrounding the nasal cavity known as sinuses. These are usually filled up with air and help in the air-conditioning of the nose and surrounding areas. Some people with dust allergy develop infection of these sinuses known as sinusitis. They complain of headache in the frontal region and pain and pressure in the face. If not treated, fever and yellow foul-smelling discharge may start dripping from the nose. This discharge may also enter the throat and cause sore throat with cough and fever. Sometimes the ears may be affected by infection giving rise to earache, muffled hearing and even pus from the ear. Infection of the eyes is also seen in some individuals with redness and swelling of the eyes and rarely corneal complications with visual impairment. Severe asthma may occur in some people with breathlessness, difficulty in lying down, fatigue and weakness, and low blood pressure.

Food Allergy

Sometimes, in sensitive individuals, food items such as peanuts, pistachios, cashewnuts, walnuts, egg-white, milk, mustard seeds, shellfish, etc. can give rise to collapse of lungs and heart, and even death.

Drug Allergy

Sometimes can be serious affecting the lungs, heart, kidney and brain and may produce near-fatal or fatal reactions. Latex allergy can also be sometimes fatal in sensitive individuals.

Insect Bite

On the tongue or mouth can be very dangerous causing compression of the airway, with tightness in the chest, breathing problem and cough, which may occur in 50-60% of patients. Giddiness and unconsciousness may occur in 30% of adults, and sometimes even death.

Skin Allergy

Patients with atopic dermatitis are prone to develop infections by bacteria, viruses and fungi. Eyes are often involved and sometimes may cause corneal deformity and cataracts.

Pet Allergy

People with pet allergy can develop a severe attack of asthma when they try to groom, dust, vacuum or clean the pet's litter box. If the cat or dog sleeps on the bed or pillows along with its master during the night, the reaction may be worse late at night or in the morning.

••

6

Effects of Seasonal Changes on Allergy

C limate plays a large role in causing allergy. The interaction of temperature, humidity and barometric pressure is important in causing or increasing the symptoms of allergy. It appears that allergic diseases, especially asthma, tend to be adversely affected by high humidity, by sudden temperature changes (particularly from warm to cold) and by drops in the barometric pressure.

Dust allergy is usually influenced by the season in which the trees pollinate, which causes the allergic pollen grains to be produced. Windy days are responsible for making the pollen grains airborne and spreading them through the environment. The susceptible individuals, on inhaling these allergens, tend to develop allergic symptoms. Dust, pollutants and other allergic elements are suspended in the atmosphere during windy and rainy days. Fungi and moulds are airborne during rainy days. Increased humidity during rainy days is also responsible for increase in allergic symptoms both in the lungs, ear, nose, throat, eyes as well as skin. Hot and humid weather is also responsible for fermentative changes in food, increase in the population of mosquitoes, houseflies and other insects which can increase incidence of **food** allergy and **insect bite** allergy.

Change of seasons from summer to winter and vice versa with changes in temperature is responsible for increase in the population of viruses which increase susceptibility to viral infections – like that of eye **(Eye-flu)**, nose **(Rhinitis)**, sinuses **(Sinusitis)** lungs **(Bronchitis)**, digestive system **(Gastroenteritis)** and skin infections **(Herpes Zoster)**.

Many symptoms of asthma will be aggravated in the cold weather as well as in the early morning hours which awakens the individuals from their sleep. Conversely, many asthmatics feel better late in the afternoon and evening hours.

Thus, change of seasons is responsible for onset of new and relapsing cases of allergies of different types.

•●

7

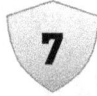

Diagnostic Tools for Detecting Allergy

S ince allergy is a very complicated and multifaceted disease, its diagnosis also involves a multipronged approach. It is based on a combination of history, signs and symptoms, laboratory tests and special tests for allergy.

The history is a fundamental part of diagnosis of allergic disease. There are certain questions that need to be asked, e.g., What are the symptoms? Do they occur in a particular place (ie. home, workplace)? Time of the day, season, after consuming certain food or medicines, after exercise, related to stress or not – are vitally important questions to be explored. Past history of same allergy or other related condition may be related to the current illness. Family history of similar allergic reactions is also significant.

Besides the history, physical examination is another equally important part of the diagnosis of allergy. It is important because there are characteristic findings of allergy which are different from non-allergic conditions but may have similar history and symptoms. Complete examination of the eyes, ears, nose, throat, lungs, skin and abdomen is essential.

The final step in making the diagnosis is done by ordering laboratory tests and investigations, which form the basis of the full and final diagnosis of allergy.

The tests which are commonly used to diagnose different types of allergies are as follows:–

❏ Blood tests
❏ Allergy testing
❏ X-rays, CT Scan, Magnetic Reasonance Imaging (MRI)
❏ Culture and Sensitivity.

Blood Tests

Among the blood tests, the important tests are the white blood cell (WBC) counts. These cells are important because they help the body in fighting against any infection as well as entry of foreign body into the system. In most of the allergies, Eosinophil, a type of WBC is increased in number in the blood.

In some cases, measurement of total immunoglobulins (Ig) in the blood is useful in differentiating the symptoms between allergic and non-allergic conditions. This is very useful in the diagnosis and treatment of the disease.

Allergy Testing

Allergy testing is usually done by two methods – skin testing and determination of allergen-specific IgE in the blood by Radio Allergosorbent Test (RAST). For skin testing, a small drop of the allergen is touched with a needle and the skin is pricked with it. In sensitive individuals, there will be redness and swelling at the site of the prick within 15 to 20 minutes. For further confirmation, a more dilute allergen is injected into the skin and looked for similar changes. In people who are very sensitive to the skin testing or are suffering from some skin disease, blood levels of allergen-specific IgE is a useful alternative. This test is also useful for detecting food allergies. It can help in detecting different types of allergens to which the person is sensitive.

X-Ray/CT Scan/MRI

Besides the above tests, X-rays, CT Scan and MRI of the nasal sinuses and lungs can help in detecting the nature of the illness. These tests help in differentiating between the allergic diseases and non-allergic ones.

Culture and Sensitivity Tests

In allergic illnesses, you can hardly find any disease-causing bacteria. This fact can be proved by taking different secretions from the nose, throat, eyes, lungs, stool, etc. and keeping them in the laboratory for 24–48 hours to observe any growth of bacteria.

These are referred to as culture and sensitivity tests. These tests help in determining the line of treatment the individual will need to overcome his illness.

●●

8

Role of Changes in Diet and Lifestyle in the Treatment

Diet and our daily activities and lifestyle have an important bearing on the symptoms and control of allergy. The conservative management of allergy includes changes in the diet and lifestyle of the individual.

Changes in the Diet

A **low-allergen** diet, also known as an **elimination diet**, is often recommended to people with suspected allergy, especially **food** allergy. It is also used as a diagnostic tool to find out if avoiding foods that commonly trigger allergies will provide relief from symptoms. In this diet, certain foods and food additives should be avoided such as wheat, milk, eggs, corn, soy, citrus fruits, nuts, peanuts, tomatoes, food preservatives and colouring agents, coffee and chocolate. This diet is maintained only until a reaction to a food substance has been diagnosed or ruled out. Once food reactions have been identified, only those foods that are causing a reaction are subsequently avoided and other foods that had previously been eaten are added to the diet. It is recommended that this low-allergen diet is followed for two weeks in order to diagnose food reactions. Strict avoidance of allergenic foods for months or years sometimes results in cessation of food allergy in some cases.

Other dietary measures to be followed are given below:–

❏ Since many individuals are allergic to proteins, a low protein diet is advised.

❏ Vegetarian diet should be preferred for easy digestion. Spicy and high calorie foods should be avoided.

❏ Eat lots of fresh green leafy vegetables.

❏ Freshly cooked food should be eaten.

❏ Fast foods, aerated drinks and alcoholic beverages should be avoided.

❏ Fruits and vegetables should be washed properly.

❏ Hands should be thoroughly washed before cooking or eating food.

❏ Food should be taken at proper timings – three regular meals in a day.

❏ Eating outside food in hot and humid weather should be avoided since during this period, several gastrointestinal viruses are rampant and may aggravate allergy.

Changes in Lifestyle

People with **dust** allergy are advised to reduce exposure to common household allergens like dust, mould and animal dander. Certain changes, as given below, can bring about long-lasting and positive results in individuals with allergy:–

❏ Minimise or give up completely usage of tea, coffee, tobacco and alcohol.

❏ Housewives should switch on their exhaust fans or use indoor chimneys while cooking food, especially while deep frying.

❏ Proper personal and household hygiene should be maintained to avoid exposure to rodents, cockroaches, insects, rats and household pests.

❏ Regular cleaning and vacuuming of rugs, carpets, curtains, furnitures, mattresses, etc., to remove dust mites is essential.

- Pets should be bathed and cleaned regularly and vacuuming of their kennels and rooms done.
- People with **dust** allergy should avoid travelling or be protected against dust-allergens on windy or rainy days.
- Avoid travelling or strolling on rainy days in parks and areas of thick vegetation to prevent insect stings and subsequent allergy.
- Certain individuals have increased work-related risks for sensitivity and exposure to latex (rubber industries), laboratory animals, biochemicals products, organic solvents, etc.

Exercise and Allergy

Though exercise is known to aggravate Bronchial Asthma in many individuals, its benefits often outweigh the adverse effects on the body. The beneficial effects brought about due to regular physical exercise are as follows:–

- Regular jogging and aerobic exercises release the muscular tension in the body, which helps in the relaxation of all muscles.
- The muscular relaxation in turn leads to mental relaxation because the body and mind are closely interlinked.
- Regular exercise also burns the calories, reduces body weight, strengthens the heart and lungs, increases stamina and body resistance towards diseases.
- Physical exercise tones up the gastrointestinal organs, increases digestion and absorption of food and speedy evacuation of bowels.

In conclusion, exercise is best for all individuals with allergy, but it should be avoided on rainy or humid days and when pollen and airborne allergens are rampant, and also in extremely cold weather conditions.

••

9

Conventional or Allopathic Treatment

Treatment of allergy by the modern system of medicine involves a systematic and multifaceted approach. It varies according to the type of allergy as well as the individual involved and severity of the disease. For a better understanding of the treatment, the following measures can be outlined:-

- ❏ Preventive aspects of treatment
- ❏ Anti-allergic medicines
- ❏ Steroids
- ❏ Allergy injections

Preventive Measures

As the old saying goes "Prevention is better than cure", the best form of treatment of allergy is to "nip it in the bud". This form of treatment involves avoidance of the allergens which are responsible for causing allergy. This is a very effective, economical and safe form of management with no adverse effects of medications. For this, allergy testing should be performed first to confirm the suspected allergens. Once the allergens are identified, the following measures can be taken for the prevention of further episodes of allergy.

- Those who are allergic to plant pollens or seasonal moulds should avoid outdoor activity during peak pollen hours, i.e., late mornings to early afternoons (11 a.m to 3 p.m). In Indian conditions hot, humid and windy days are bad for people with dust allergy.

- For those who are allergic to grass pollens, wearing a surgical type mask while mowing the lawn or gardening may help in averting symptoms of allergy.

- Keeping the windows closed throughout the day and using an airconditioner can prevent airborne pollens from entering indoors.

- To prevent house dust-mite allergy, specially constructed pillow, mattress and box-spring covers made of fabrics or plastics that act as a barrier for allergens should be used.

- All sheets, mattress pads, pillow cases and blankets should be washed every week in hot water to kill the dust mites.

- The carpets may be removed or treated with tannic acid spray or vacuumed frequently with vacuum cleaners with attached filters.

- For prevention of pet allergy, the animal should be kept outside the house and the carpet and all rooms should be thoroughly cleaned.

- To avoid presence of indoor fungi and moulds like Aspergillus, Penicillium and Alternaria, leaky roofs, ceilings, flooded basements and damaged plumbing should be repaired. Dehumidifiers are also useful.

- Extermination of household pests like cockroaches, mosquitoes, houseflies, rats, etc., is essential. Traps, bait and hygiene control are necessary but sprays may aggravate asthma.

- The mainstay of treatment of skin, insect, drug and food allergy is discontinuation of contact with the offending agent. Thus, the identification and avoidance of the allergic substance remains the key to resolve the problem. Careful education should be provided regarding sources of the allergen and how to avoid it.

❏ Educating the person as well as the family members is a useful measure in controlling different types of allergies. In case of food allergy, when eating out, the contents of the prepared food should be enquired. At home even, warning stickers should be placed on foods with the offending antigen for food-sensitive individuals.

Anti-allergic Medicines

Depending on the type, there are several medications for treatment and control of allergy. They are as follows:–

❏ Antihistamines
❏ Medicines for asthma
❏ Antibiotics
❏ Local (topical) agents

Antihistamines

In the process of allergy, certain chemical substances called mediators are released from the body. Of these, the most important mediator is known as **Histamine.**

The basic medical treatment of allergy lies in reducing the effects of histamine, i.e. sneezing, itching, running nose, breathing problems, swelling of the skin, nose, lungs, etc. Most of the histamine effects occur when histamine binds to the affected tissues or organs via histamine receptors. There are three types of histamine receptors (H1, H_2 and H_3) of which H_1 receptors are most important. A list of commonly used antihistamines is given for easy reference.

Commonly Used Antihistamines

Pharmacological Name	Popular Brand Name
Pheniramine maleate	Avil
Chlorpheniramine maleate	Cadistin
Dexchlorpheniramine maleate	Polaramine
Diphenhydramine	Benadryl
Cyproheptadine	Practin
Dimethindene maleate	Foristal
Embramine	Mebryl
Azatadine maleate	Zadine
Astemizole	Stemiz
Terfenadine	Trexyl
Cetirizine	Alerid
Levocetirizine	Levorid
Clemastine fumarate	Tavegyl
Loratadine	Loridin
Hydroxyzine	Atarax
Methdilazine	Dilosyn
Desloratadine	Deslor
Fexofenadine	Allegra
Ebastine	Ebast
Ketotifen	Ketasma
Mizolastine	Elina
Flunisolide	Syntaris (spray)
Azelastine	Azep (spray)

These antihistamines are quite successful in controlling the main and early symptoms of allergy but they have certain side-effects. The usual adverse effects are headache, drowsiness, giddiness, dryness of the mouth, blurring of vision, diarrhoea, stomach-ache, flatulence (gas) and fatigue. The adverse effects are lesser with newer antihistamines like Cetirizine, Fexofenadine, Joratadine, Azelastine, etc.

Medicines for Asthma

Asthma is a disease associated with narrowed breathing pathways which leads to spells of breathlessness, giddiness, cough, noisy breathing and other symptoms. There are several medicines which are used in controlling Bronchial Asthma. A list of medicines with their popular brand names is given below:–

Commonly Used Medicines for Asthma

Pharmacological Name	Brand Name
Salbutamol	Asthalin, Ventorlin
Theophylin + Etophylin	Deriphylin
Terbutaline	Bricanyl
Bambuterol	Bambudil
Ketotifen	Asthafen, Ketasma
Montelukast	Emlucast, Ventair
Zaferlukot	Zuvair

Mechanisms of action of the above medicines are as follows:–

❏ Improve functioning of the lungs by bronchodilatation (increasing elasticity).

❏ Decrease number of eosinophils in the blood which are responsible for the allergy.

❏ Remove mucus and dust from the lungs.

❏ Facilitate easy breathing.

❏ Control the symptoms of allergy.

❏ Prevent symptoms of asthma and allergy following exercise or due to intake of painkillers like aspirin.

❏ Improve symptoms of allergy in the nose and sinuses.

Antibiotics

In almost all types of allergy, there is a superadded infection in the due course of time. This is due to the entry of bacteria in these areas. Depending on the condition and the type of bacteria, the antibiotic is selected and needs to be given for a period ranging from one week to six weeks. The commonly used antibiotics are Amoxycillin, Septran, Clarithromycin, Azithromycin, Cefuroxime, Levofloxacin, Cefixime, Cefpodoxime, Clindamycin, etc.

Local (topical) Agents

In the treatment of allergy, certain medicines are directly applied at the affected site for early and better results. These are known as local or topical agents. They come in the form of nasal drops and sprays, inhalers, eye drops and ointments, skin creams, lotions, etc. A list of some of the popular brands of topical agents is given in the table below:–

Popular Local (Topical) Agents

Nasal drops/ sprays	Inhalers	Eye drops/ ointments	Skin Creams
Otrivin	Asthalin	Locula	Neosporin
Dristan	Beclate	Cifran	Betadine
Endrine	Bricanyl	Genticyn	Furacin
Ifiral	Budecort	Chloromycetin	Flucort
Flomist	Foracort	Ensamycin	Betnovate
Efcorlin	Metaspray	Silverex	Clobate

Role of Steroids in Allergy

Steroids or corticosteroids are currently the most important class of medicines used to treat allergy. The mechanism of action of steroids by which they combat allergy are as given on the next page:–

46

- By modulating the function of white blood cells in order to minimise the symptoms of allergy.
- By inhibiting production of chemical mediators which cause allergy.
- By reducing mucus secretion in the airways.
- By decreasing inflammation of the airways and improving aeration.

Corticosteroids are available in different forms as oral medicines, injections, nasal drops/sprays, inhalers, eye drops, skin creams, etc.

Some of the popular brands of steroids are Wysolone, Betnesol, Decadron, Cortisone, Kenacort, etc.

The steroids are wonderful medicines except for their side-effects which include weight gain, high blood pressure, ulcers in the stomach, cataracts, softening of bones, stunting of growth, psychological changes and aggravation of diabetes. However, these side-effects only occur after prolonged use of these medicines.

Allergy Injections

Some people who do not respond to the above measures may benefit from allergy injections also known as allergen immunotherapy. The candidates for this therapy are as follows:-

- Those who do not respond to allergen avoidance.
- Those who do not respond to anti-allergic medicine.
- Those who develop severe side-effects of medicines.
- Those who cannot adhere to complex regimen of multiple medications.
- Those who suffer from multiple allergies.

The basic concept or goal of allergy injections is to help the body in producing more of immunoglobulin (Ig)G to counterbalance the excessive levels of immunoglobulin (Ig)E which are common in allergic individuals.

In this method, the doctor injects a serum containing allergenic substances such as dust, pollen, animal dander, food extract, etc., just below the skin surface. The cells that make IgE antibodies are located on the skin surface while the cells that make IgG antibodies are located in the liver, lymph nodes and spleen. This method bypasses the skin surface and the serum enters the body to produce IgG instead of IgE.

These injections are given in increasing doses once or twice a week for two to three months and then once a month for two to three years. About 80% of people experience improvement after one to two years and the effects persist for several years. People with **dust** allergy benefit the most from this treatment.

●●

10

Does Yoga have an Answer to this Problem

What is Yoga

Yoga is an ancient Indian technique of integrating human personality at the physical, mental, moral and intellectual levels.

Maharishi Patanjali explained Yoga as *Chitta Vritti Nirodha* or control of the mind and all its fluctuations. He described eight aspects (limbs) of Yoga which may be used to attain a healthy, happy and spiritual life. These are as follows:–

1. "Yama" or moral principles like non-violence, truthfulness, honesty, celibacy and non-covetousness.

2. "Niyama" or rules of discipline like purity, contentment, austerity, introspection and dedication to God.

3. "Asanas" or yogic postures.

4. "Pranayama" or control of breathing.

5. "Pratyahara" or control of the mind and the sense organs.

6. "Dharana" or concentration.

7. "Dhyana" or meditation.

8. "Samadhi" or a state of transcendental consciousness when the individual merges with the universal spirit.

Role of Yoga in the Treatment of Allergy

From the treatment point of view, Yoga can be divided as follows:-

❑ Yogasanas
❑ Yogic Kriyas
❑ Pranayama
❑ Meditation

Yogasanas

Yogasanas refer to the yogic postures of the body, which help in the physical, mental and spiritual development of the individual.

Difference between Physical Exercise & Yogasanas

S. No.		Physical Exercise	Yogasanas
1.	Movement of body	Moves rapidly.	Moves slowly and uniformly.
2.	Age groups	Restrictions are present in different age groups, especially older people.	Can be practised by male, female and aged persons.
3.	Good effect on body	Strengthens the muscles.	Strengthens the mind and also the muscles.
4.	Outcome	Causes anxiety, exhaustion and weariness.	Tones up the nerves and internal organs of body. Exhaustion and weariness is not felt.
5.	Development of body and mind	Mainly assists in development of body.	Develops body, mind and prana.
6.	Flexibility of body	Lesser	More

S. No.		Physical Exercise	Yogasanas
7.	Discontinuation	Cannot be given up suddenly.	Can be discontinued at any time.
8.	Diet	Very rich food is required.	Simple and pure food.
9.	Prevention and cure of disease	Prevention possible. Cure not available.	Have such powers.

How do Yogasanas Help in the Treatment of Allergy

❑ All abdominal organs are toned up and the digestion and metabolism of food substances are enhanced.

❑ Better metabolism helps in digesting even the allergic or indigestible substances with ease.

❑ There is a proper conditioning and rejuvenation of the neuro-endocrine (hormonal) system.

❑ The immune system is activated enabling the body to withstand greater stress and strain, including that due to allergy.

❑ Accumulated toxic substances and allergic products are easily eliminated keeping the body fit, strong and rejuvenated.

❑ Regular practice of Yogasanas helps to voluntarily control the heart rate, respiration, excretion, body temperature, requirement of food, sleep, etc., bringing about a state of economical self-preservation and conservation of energy.

Yogasanas Useful for Treatment of Allergy

In individuals with **dust** allergy and **skin** allergy, the following asanas are beneficial:

Dhanurasana, Paschimottanasana, Sarvangasana, Bhujangasana, Naukasana, Matsyasana, Pawan Muktasana, Simhasana, Trikonasana and Surya Namaskar.

For individuals with **food** allergy the useful Yogasanas are *Surya Namaskar, Pawan Muktasana, Trikonasana, Halasana, Tadasana, Ardhamatsyendrasana, Shashankasana, Kati Chakrasana, Matsyasana,* and *Bhujangasana.*

Detailed descriptions of certain important asanas are given below:–

Dhanurasana (Bow Pose)

Technique

❏ Lie down in the prone position (on the stomach) with the face and forehead touching the ground with the legs straight and the arms by the side.

❏ Exhale and bend the legs at the knee and hold them firmly by the hands at the ankles on the same side.

❏ Inhale, raise the thighs, chest and head simultaneously.

❏ The weight of the body should be on the navel and the head should be raised as high as possible with eyes looking upwards.

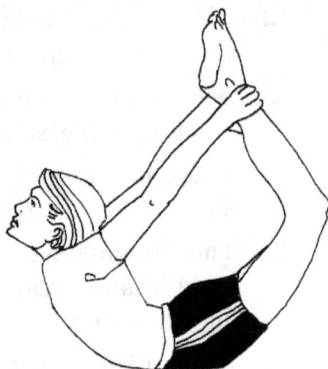

Fig. Dhanurasana

❏ This posture should be held as long as it is felt comfortable.

❏ Some authors recommend mild rocking movement on the abdomen, which bears the weight.

❏ Repeat this 3-5 times.

Precautions

❏ This asana should not be done by those suffering from high blood pressure, slipped disc, hernia, colitis, duodenal ulcer and heart diseases.

Paschimottanasana *(Back Stretching Pose)*

Technique

❑ Sit on the floor with the legs outstretched, feet together and hands on the knees.

❑ Relaxing the whole body slowly bend forward from the hips, sliding the hands down the legs. Try to grasp the big toes with the fingers and thumbs. If not possible hold the heels, ankles or any part of the legs that can be reached comfortably.

❑ Hold this position for a few seconds.

❑ Keep the legs straight, bend the elbows and gently bring the trunk down towards the legs keeping a firm grip on the toes, feet or legs. Touch the knees with the forehead and hold in this position as long as it is comfortable.

❑ Slowly return to the original position.

❑ Relax and repeat the exercise 2-3 times.

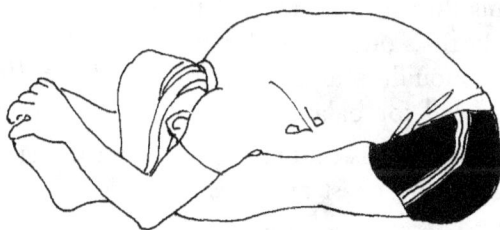

Fig. Paschimottanasana

Precautions

❑ People who suffer from slipped disc, lumbar spondylitis or sciatica should not perform this asana.

❑ Similarly, those with cardiac problems, hernia and those who have undergone abdominal surgery should avoid this asana.

Sarvangasana (Shoulder Stand)

It is a core exercise for all practitioners of Yoga and sometimes called as "the mother of all asanas".

Technique

❏ Lie down in a supine position with legs and arms straight, feet together and palms facing downward.

❏ Take a deep breath and lift both the legs slowly upwards till they are at right angle to the body.

❏ After exhaling, pause for a few seconds.

❏ Inhale and lift legs, buttocks and lower back with the forearms so that the chin presses into the sternum. Thus the entire weight of the body rests on the head, neck and shoulders and the arms are used for balancing.

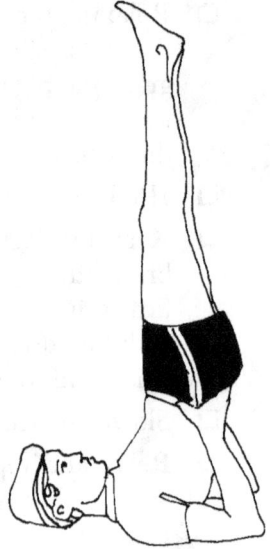

Fig. Sarvangasana

❏ Focus the eyes on the big toes with the chin pressed against the chest and breathe slowly.

❏ Maintain this posture for 2-3 minutes.

❏ Exhale and bring down the legs after releasing the hands and the palms.

Precautions

❏ This asana should not be practised by individuals with high blood pressure, heart disease, cervical spondylitis and slipped disc.

❏ Obese individuals, people with a weak backbone or abdominal muscles and beginners are advised to support their legs against a wall initially.

□ It should be avoided during menstruation and advanced pregnancy.

Bhujangasana (Serpent Pose)

Technique

□ Lie flat on the ground in the prone position with legs straight, feet extended and touching each other, and forehead pressed to the ground.

□ Breathe in, press the head back and slowly raise the head and shoulders off the ground by bending the neck and back muscles.

□ Keeping the arms straight, lift the abdomen above the navel from the ground with the head looking upwards into the sky.

□ Hold your breath and remain in the posture for a few seconds with the weight of the body balanced by the arms.

□ Slowly exhale and come back to the original position. Repeat the process 2-3 times.

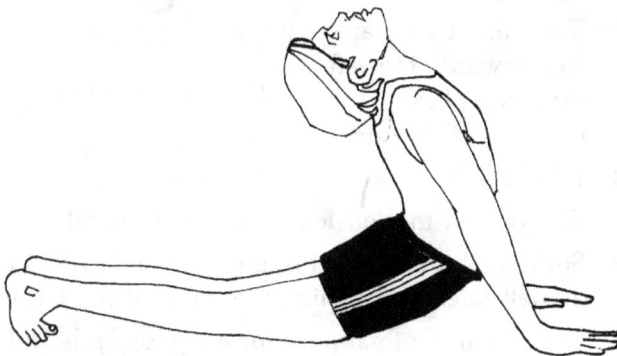

Fig. Bhujangasana

Precautions

□ Individuals who suffer from hypertension, peptic ulcer, hernia, intestinal TB, and hyperthyroidism should not practise this asana.

Ardhamatsyendrasana
(Spinal Twist Pose)

This asana is a very important one since it strengthens the flexibility of spine laterally (sideways) which no other asana can accomplish. It is a very useful asana for patients prone to allergy.

Technique

❏ Sit on the floor with the legs extended in front and feet together.

❏ Bend the right knee and bring the heel of the right foot close to the left buttock.

❏ Now bend the left knee and place the foot on the outer surface of the right hip.

❏ Turn the trunk and face towards the left shoulder placing the left arm behind the back.

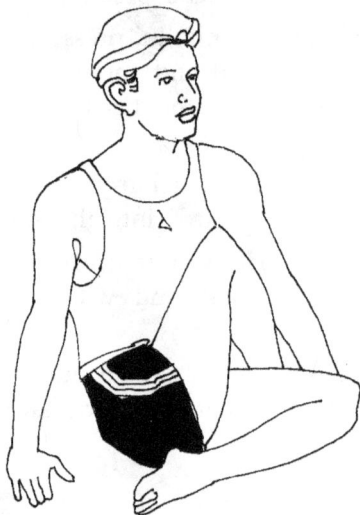

Fig : Ardhamatsyendrasana

❏ Hold the left ankle with the right hand.

❏ Try to hold the left leg with the left hand.

❏ Some authors advise bringing the right hand under the left knee and joining the palm of the left hand.

❏ Remain in the final pose for a few seconds and then return to the original position.

❏ Repeat the same with the other side.

Precautions

❏ This asana should be done slowly and steadily without exerting undue pressure on the spine.

- People with peptic ulcer, hernia, hyperthyroidism, sciatica, and pregnant women, should practise this asana only under expert guidance.

Matsyasana (Fish Pose)

This asana is called Matsyasana because it is said that yogis could float on water like fishes while in this asana, by holding their breath.

Technique

- Assume a sitting position with the legs bent at the knees and the feet kept on opposite hip joints. The heels are adjusted in such a way that each presses the adjacent portion of the abdomen. This forms a foot-lock as in Padmasana.
- Bend backwards with the head resting on the crown and the weight of the body on the elbows.

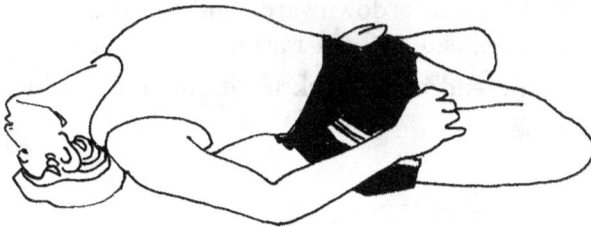

Fig. Matsyasana

- Push the neck backwards enhancing forcibly and slightly raise the hip and chest upwards thus making an arch of the spine.
- Hold the toes on the corresponding side by hooking the fingers.
- Breathe deeply and stay in this position as long as possible.
- Then release the neck and let the head rest on the floor. Straighten the legs and relax the hands, elbows and the whole body.

❏ Repeat the asana, with the legs crossed the other way.

Precautions

The arching of the spine should be done slowly to avoid injury to spine.

Shashankasana (Hare Pose)

Technique

❏ Sit with legs folded backwards, heels apart, knees and toes together. (Vajrasana)
❏ Let both the hips fit in between the heels.
❏ Inhale and slowly raise the arms over the head.
❏ While exhaling, slowly bend forward, resting the palms on the floor and the abdomen pressing against the thighs.
❏ Bring the face downwards and touch the floor with the forehead without raising the buttocks.
❏ Inhale and come back to the original position.
❏ Repeat 3-5 times.

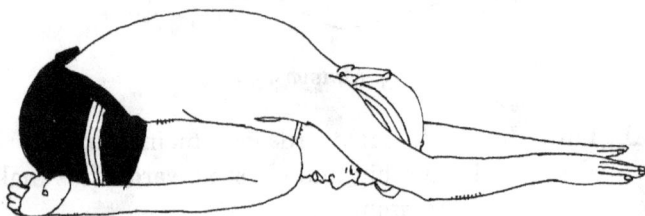

Fig. Shashankasana

Precautions

❏ This exercise should not be done by persons suffering from cervical spondylitis, lumbar spondylitis, vertigo and hypertension.

Yogic Kriyas

Yogic Kriyas are a very important part of Hatha Yoga as they help to eliminate the accumulated toxins from the body. The body is like a machine, which has to be continuously cleaned and maintained in a perfect condition. The Yogic Kriyas are six in number and often referred to as Shat Kriyas. They are as follows:–

❑ Neti
❑ Kapalbhati
❑ Dhauti
❑ Nauli
❑ Basti
❑ Trataka

Kriyas useful for treatment of allergy are Kapalbhati, Neti, and Vaman Dhauti (Kunjal Kriya).

How Yogic Kriyas help in Allergy

❑ They help in cleansing the body of toxins like the allergens, mucus, gas, acid, sweat, urine and stool.

❑ They improve the functioning of the excretory organs.

❑ They help keep the eyes, nose, sinuses, respiratory and digestive systems clean and tone up their functioning.

❑ These Kriyas help to build up resistance to diseases and sharpen the mind.

❑ They also help to prepare the body and condition it for proper practice of Yogasanas, Yoga Nidra, pranayama and meditation.

❑ If done regularly these techniques are capable of curing different types of allergies.

Kapalbhati (Frontal Brain Cleansing)

Kapalbhati is basically a technique of pranayama though older yogic texts have classified it as a part of Shatkarmas. It is of three types: Vatkrama Kapalbhati, Vyutkrama Kapalbhati and Sheetkrama Kapalbhati.

Vatkrama Kapalbhati

This is the most beneficial technique for treatment of allergy.

Technique

- ❑ Sit in any comfortable asana with the head and spine straight and the hands resting on the knees.
- ❑ Close the eyes and relax the whole body.
- ❑ Inhale deeply through both nostrils expanding the abdomen and exhale with a forceful contraction of the abdominal muscles, making a hissing noise.
- ❑ The next inhalation takes place by passively allowing the abdominal muscles to expand spontaneously without any effort.
- ❑ After completing 10 rapid breaths in succession, inhale and exhale deeply completing one round.
- ❑ Complete 3-5 such rounds.

Precautions

- ❑ The rapid breathing in this technique should be from the abdomen and not from the chest.
- ❑ It should be practised after asanas or Neti and preferably on an empty stomach or 3-4 hours after meals.
- ❑ If pain or giddiness is experienced, it should be stopped for a while and continued.
- ❑ Kapalbhati should not be practised by those suffering from heart disease, high blood pressure, vertigo, epilepsy, stroke, hernia or peptic ulcer.

Vaman Dhauti or Kunjal Kriya

Technique

- ❑ Take about 1 litre of lukewarm water flavoured with aniseed and cardamom, to which some salt is added.

- Drink this water as quickly as possible till a vomiting sensation is felt.
- Stand up immediately, bend forward and insert first 3 fingers of the right hand into the mouth and tickle the uvula till vomiting is induced.
- Continue this process till all the water comes out.
- This can be repeated once a week.

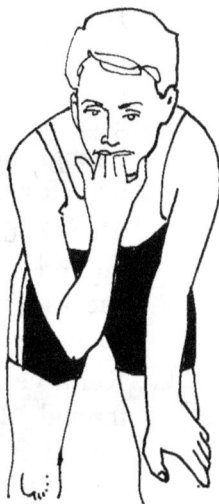

Kunjal Kriya or Vaman Dhauti

Precautions

- This procedure should be done in the early morning on an empty stomach.
- Food should not be taken for at least half an hour after practice.
- Fingernails should be trimmed well and hands washed with soap and water before performing the procedure.
- Persons suffering from stomach ulcers, eye diseases, heart problems, stroke, hernia should avoid this kriya.

Neti

Neti is a process that helps to clean the nasal passages. This is of three types:-
- Sutraneti or Rubberneti
- Jalaneti
- Ghrithaneti or Ghee drops

Sutraneti or Rubberneti

Technique

- A cotton string stiffened with wax or a rubber catheter of numbers 3,4 or 5 is used.

- It is slowly inserted through one nostril with the right hand and gradually pulled out through the mouth with the left hand.
- Then both the ends are moved forwards and backwards in the nostril about 15-20 times.
- Remove the string through the mouth and repeat the same procedure for the other nostril.

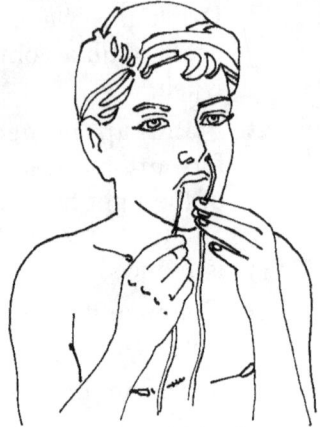

Fig. Sutraneti

- This procedure is done once daily initially and after one month reduced to twice or thrice a week.

Precautions

- This procedure is to be strictly done under the guidance of an expert.
- Persons with high blood pressure, bleeding from nose, deviated nasal septum and severe cold should not practise this kriya.
- Fingernails should be properly cut and hands washed with soap and water.
- Spectacles if any should be removed before practising Neti.
- In the beginning of Neti, when the thread or catheter is introduced, there may be an itching sensation in the nostrils with sneezing and watering from the eyes. These symptoms will subside with regular practice.

Jalaneti

This is another technique of nasal cleansing using salt water instead of thread or catheter.

Technique

- Boil about a litre of water in a vessel and allow it to cool.

- Add a teaspoonful of salt to it and stir well.

- Transfer this water to a Jalaneti pot.

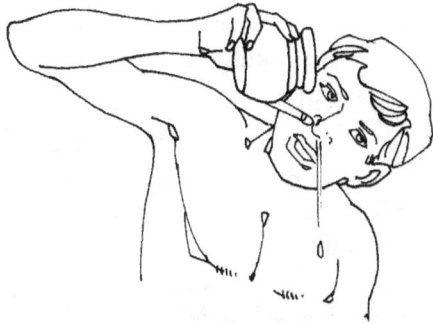

Fig. Jalaneti

- Stand erect, stoop forward and insert the spout gently into one of the nostrils.

- Slowly tilt the head to the other side so that water runs into one nostril and comes out of the other.

- Keep the mouth open and breathe normally through the mouth.

- Allow water to flow freely through the other nostril continuously like a stream.

- Repeat the procedure for the other nostril.

- This procedure should be done once daily or more often if one is suffering from cold and stuffy nose.

Precautions

- The concentration of salt and the temperature of water should be maintained throughout the practice.

- The nozzle of Jalaneti pot should not be inserted too deeply into the nostril since it may injure the sensitive lining of the nose.

- Do not inhale through the nose or else the salt water will enter the mouth.

- In the beginning of the procedure there may be itching or irritation in the nose, sneezing or watering of the eyes. This will improve with practice.

- ❏ The nose should be dried properly after the procedure since water left off may cause cold and sinusitis. This can be done by moving the head in different directions and exhaling forcibly.
- ❏ This procedure should not be done after meals.
- ❏ Do not blow the nose too hard since the water may be pushed into the ears.

Ghrithaneti

Technique

Pure desi ghee prepared from cow's milk is applied in the form of nasal drops. This ghee is to be warmed until it liquefies and then with the help of a dropper 1-2 drops of it is applied into each nostril. After applying ghee, cover the face with a towel and rub the area around the nose. Ghrithaneti should be done before doing Sutraneti and Jalaneti.

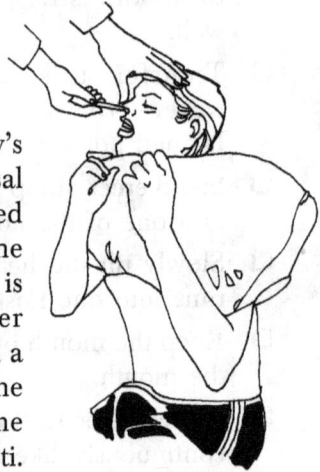

Fig. Ghrithaneti

Pranayama

Pranayama is derived from two Sanskrit words – "Prana" and "Ayama". "Prana" means breath, life, vitality, air, power or energy. "Ayama" denotes extension, abstinence, regulation, control or restraint. Thus Pranayama is the act of control of respiration and an attempt to control the flow of "Prana" or vital force in the human body.

Stages of Pranayama

Pranayama consists of four stages:–

- ❏ The "Puraka" or Inhalation Phase: Long, slowly controlled and sustained flow of inhalation.
- ❏ The "Kumbhaka" or Breath-holding phase: Controlled suspension and retention of breath after inhalation.

- The "Rechaka" or Exhalation Phase: Long, slow and controlled exhalation.
- "Shunyaka" or End of Breathing: Breath-holding after exhalation.

Benefits of Pranayama in Allergy

- Pranayama combats and cures allergy by cleansing the nose, nasal sinuses and respiratory passages of allergic substances like pollen, dust and other toxic substances.
- Pranayama improves the function of the lungs by increased oxygenation of blood vessels of the lungs as well as all parts of the body.
- It increases the capacity of the lungs to inhale and exhale air.
- Breath-holding can train the body to tolerate low oxygen levels as seen while climbing the mountains.
- The blood supply to the heart and brain is improved by Pranayama.
- It enhances the concentration of mind and improves the relaxation of the body.
- The digestive system is toned up due to improved blood supply and pressure of the diaphragm on the abdominal organs. This is very beneficial for all individuals with **food** allergy. Moreover, the toxic substances are removed from the digestive tract.

Pranayama Useful for Treatment of Allergy

Nadi Shodhana Pranayama or Anuloma Viloma, Bhastrika, Suryabhedi and Ujjayi are very beneficial for treatment of allergy and produce long-lasting results.

Nadi Shodhana Pranayama or Anuloma-Viloma

Technique

- Sit in any comfortable meditative posture, preferably Padmasana, keeping the head and spine upright.

- Close the eyes, relax the body and breathe freely for some time.
- Rest the index and middle fingers gently in the centre of eyebrows, and the thumb and ring finger above the right and left nostrils respectively. These two fingers control the flow of breath in the nostrils by alternately pressing on one nostril and blocking the flow of breath and then the other. This is the Nasikagra Mudra.

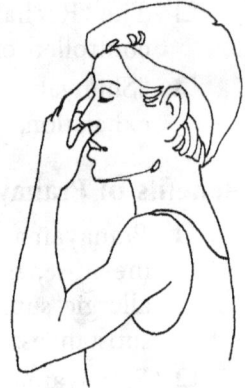

Fig. Nadi Shodhana Pranayama

Step–I

- Close the right nostril with the thumb and breathe in through the left nostril, mentally counting 1,2,3. Similarly, close the left nostril with the ring finger, releasing pressure of thumb on the right nostril and breathe out, mentally counting 1,2,3. The time for inhalation and exhalation should be equal.
- Repeat the procedure by inhaling through the right nostril and exhaling through the left one. This makes up one round. Ten rounds are to be practised.
- Slowly increase the counting up to 12:12 for inhalation/exhalation. This is followed by changing the ratio to 1:2, i.e., breathe in for count 5 and breathe out for count 10 adding up to ratio 12:24.

Step–II

After mastering step I, this step should be practised:-

- Close the right nostril and inhale through the left nostril for a count of 5. After this, close both nostrils and retain air in the lungs for a count of 5. Then, open the right nostril, breathe in slightly and slowly breathe out for a count of 5.

- ❏ This is repeated by inhaling from the right nostril, retaining and breathing out from the left side. Repeat 10 rounds.
- ❏ Increase the ratio from 1:1:1 for inhalation, retention and exhalation to 1:1:2, then 1:2:2, 1:3:2 and 1:4:2.

Step-III

- ❏ In this step, inhalation is started from the left nostril as above, followed by retention (breath-holding) and exhalation from right nostril, which is also followed by breath-holding.
- ❏ The procedure is also repeated as above by inhalation from the right nostril and 10 rounds are completed.
- ❏ The ratio is started as above 1:1:1:1 and increased to 1:4:2:2 and duration is also increased from a count of 5 to the maximum limit where comfortable.

Precautions

- ❏ Breathing should be free flowing and never forced.
- ❏ Breathing should never be done through the mouth.
- ❏ This technique of Pranayama is best done under the guidance of an expert.
- ❏ If there is any sign of discomfort, the procedure should be discontinued.
- ❏ The best time to practise is early in the morning after the asanas.
- ❏ The duration of this Pranayama should be about 10-15 minutes daily comprising 5-10 rounds.
- ❏ Patients suffering from hypertension and heart disease must avoid breath-holding in this Pranayama.

Bhastrika Pranayama

Technique

- ❏ Sit in any comfortable meditative posture with hands resting on the knees in Gyana Mudra.

- ❏ Keep the head and spine straight, close the eyes and relax the whole body.
- ❏ Using Nasikagra Mudra close the right nostril with the thumb.
- ❏ Breathe in and out forcefully, without straining through the left nostril, about 10 times. The abdomen should expand and contract rhythmically with the breath.
- ❏ Now close the left nostril and breathe rapidly and forcefully through the right nostril.
- ❏ Similarly, breathing can be done through both the nostrils simultaneously.
- ❏ At the end of each procedure, breath-holding may be done for up to 30 seconds.

Precautions

- ❏ During Bhastrika, only the abdomen should move and not the chest or shoulders.
- ❏ The breathing sound should only appear from the abdomen and not the throat or chest.
- ❏ If there is a feeling of giddiness, vomiting or excessive perspiration, Bhastrika should be stopped.
- ❏ Violent respiration, facial contortions and excessive shaking of the body should be avoided.
- ❏ Bhastrika should not be practised by people suffering from hypertension, heart disease, duodenal ulcer, hernia, stroke, epilepsy or vertigo.
- ❏ Neti may be practised if there is blockage of nostrils with mucus.

Ujjayi Pranayama

Technique

- ❏ Sit in any comfortable meditative posture.
- ❏ Close the eyes and relax the whole body.

- Inhale slowly and deeply through both the nostrils with a low, uniform frictional sound through the glottis and expand the chest naturally.
- Hold the breath for some time.
- Then exhale through both the nostrils.
- Relax the chest for a few seconds after going into the next round.
- Practise for 10-20 minutes.

Precautions

- Care should be taken to see that the abdomen does not bulge out during inspiration.
- Breath-holding should not be done by patients of heart disease.
- Do not contract the throat or facial muscles strongly.
- People with spondylitis or slipped disc can practise it in Vajrasana or Makarasana.

Meditation

Patanjali, the original teacher of Yoga had described meditation as "the uninterrupted thinking of one thought". Swami Vivekananda had said, "Meditation is the focussing of the mind on some object. If the mind acquires concentration on one object, it can concentrate on any object whatsoever."

Basic Procedure of Meditation

Though different religions, communities and sects may have some variation in the procedure of meditation, the basic procedure is almost similar in all cases. The main goal in meditation is to withdraw the mind and senses from the surrounding environment and focus the attention on any given object.

Meditation is usually done in the following steps:–

Complete Relaxation

Complete relaxation refers to conscious suspension of all movements of the body resulting in relaxation of all skeletal muscles and limpness of the body.

❏ Adopt either sitting postures like Padmasana, Sukhasana and Vajrasana or the standing posture.

❏ Maintain the posture and keep the spine and neck straight and the whole body relaxed.

❏ Concentrate your mind on each part of the body one by one, starting from the toes to the head.

❏ Allow each part to relax and feel that it has become relaxed completely.

Awareness of Breathing

❏ Concentrate completely on the breathing, taking slow deep and rhythmic breaths.

❏ Concentrate at the meeting point of both nasal cavities and perceive both the incoming and outgoing breaths.

❏ Next concentrate on the navel and be fully aware of the contraction and expansion of abdominal muscles during exhalation and inhalation respectively.

❏ Alternate breathing can also be practised during meditation without causing any wandering thoughts or discomfort.

Awareness of Body Parts

❏ Concentrate on each part of the body one by one, perceiving the sensations and vibrations in each part. Start with the big toe of right foot, moving upwards in the front and back to the head, focussing on each part.

❏ Perceive the body as a whole while assuming or even standing up slowly from the sitting posture.

70

Awareness of Chakras or Psychic Centres

❏ While sitting in the relaxed posture, focus the attention on the seven chakras or psychic centres, starting from the Muladhara Chakra or Shakti Kendra.

❏ Imagine as if the vibrations are flowing from Muladhara Chakra upwards up to Sahasra Chakra or Jyoti Kendra.

S. No.	Chakra/Psychic Centre	Location	Corresponding Organ
1.	Muladhara Chakra or Shakti Kendra (centre of energy.)	Lower end of spinal cord and genitals.	Gonads-testes/ovaries.
2.	Swadhisthana Chakra or Taijasa Kendra (centre of bioelectricity.)	Below navel and back.	Adrenals, Spleen.
3.	Manipura Chakra.	Above navel and back.	Pancreas and liver.
4.	Anahata Chakra or Ananda Kendra (centre of bliss.)	Chest and heart region.	Thymus.
5.	Vishuddi Chakra/Kendra (centre of purity).	Throat and back of neck.	Thyroid and parathyroid glands.
6.	Ajna Chakra or Darshan Kendra (centre of intuition.)	Centre of eyebrows.	Pituitary gland.
7.	Sahasra Chakra or Jyoti Kendra (centre of enlightenment).	Top of head.	Pineal gland.

Awareness of Psychic Colours

The chakras or psychic centres can be activated by visualising certain colours, which are capable of producing specific vibrations. This is possible by regular practice of meditation.

While perceiving the different chakras or psychic centres, one should visualise a particular colour, which is specific for it (refer Table below). This helps in activating these centres and enhancing their physiological functions.

S. No.	Chakra/Psychic Centre	Colour to be Visualised
1.	Muladhara Chakra or Shakti Kendra.	Red
2.	Swadhisthana Chakra or Taijasa Kendra.	Orange
3.	Manipura Chakra.	Yellow
4.	Anahata Chakra or Ananda Kendra.	Green
5.	Vishuddhi Chakra/Kendra.	Blue
6.	Ajna Chakra or Darshan Kendra.	Purple
7.	Sahasra Chakra or Jyoti Kendra.	White

Auto-Suggestion and Resolution

Auto-suggestion refers to repeated recitation of a sentence, e.g., "The pain in my knee is disappearing," or "My headache has gone," etc. Auto-suggestion helps in building up faith and belief and the tolerance to bear the disease or its effects. This also brings up physiological changes in the body, weakening the forces of disease, mental imbalance and emotional disturbances.

Resolution or contemplation refers to building up healthy and positive attitude towards life. This can be done by repeating "I will not steal," or "I will tell the truth," or "I will stand first in the class," etc. Repetition of such a resolution helps in overcoming negative attitudes and psychological distortions, and develops positive attitudes like truthfulness, amity, fearlessness, tolerance, love, sympathy, etc.

Role of Meditation in the Treatment of Allergy

❏ Regular practice of meditation is capable of boosting up and modulating our immune system and controlling allergy, which is an immune disorder. Thus, even if an individual experiences an allergic reaction on being exposed to the specific allergen, the allergic response will not be so severe to affect the normal activities.

❏ For individuals with **dust** allergy, it is advisable to activate the Sahasra, Ajna, Vishuddi and Anahata Chakras by visualising the corresponding colours given in the Table. In those with **food** allergy, activation of Manipura and Swadhisthana Chakras is essential.

❏ During the phase of autosuggestion, the affected person should say repeatedly: "My allergy is controlled and I am perfectly normal." These statements help in bringing about physiological changes in the body and reducing the intensity of allergic symptoms and sometimes even lead to complete freedom from these symptoms.

❏ Regular practice of meditation stabilises and strengthens the neuro-muscular, neuro-endocrine and immunological systems keeping the body fit and free from allergy.

❏ Negative thoughts and emotions are controlled helping people to overcome stress, which may be one of the precipitating factors of allergy.

●●

11

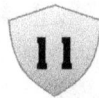

What is the Role of Naturopathy (Nature Cure)

Naturopathy or Nature Cure is the technique of following the rules of Nature and exploiting the natural resources like the sun, air, water and soil to cure the various maladies affecting man.

The branches of Naturopathy which are useful for treatment of Allergy are:-

❏ Hydrotherapy
❏ Mud Therapy
❏ Massage.

Hydrotherapy

Water is very essential for our life. It not only quenches our thirst but also has certain medicinal properties by virtue of its rich mineral content. Water contains copper, carbon, sulphur, phosphorus, iodine, calcium and other valuable minerals and chemicals of medicinal value.

How does Hydrotherapy work in Treatment of Allergy

❏ Hot water is useful in removing congestion of blood around the organs where it is applied, thereby increasing blood circulation to that area.

- Cold water will reduce swelling and inflammation, and relax the blood vessels in these areas, hence normalising the blood circulation.
- Hydrotherapy removes the sluggishness of the various organs and activates the function of digestion and metabolism.
- Accumulation of toxins and waste products in the body is eliminated.

Types of Hydrotherapy Useful for Treatment of Allergy

For Dust Allergy
- Hot/Neutral spinal bath
- Neutral spinal spray
- Heat compress on the chest
- Hot foot bath
- Alternate hot and cold bath
- Steam inhalation

For Food Allergy
- Cold spinal bath
- Cold spinal spray
- Heat compress on the abdomen
- Friction rub
- Alternate hip or revulsive hip bath
- Hot foot bath

Cold Spinal Bath
A specially designed tub called spinal bath tub is used for this bath. The side of the tub is slightly elevated so that the patient can keep his head on it comfortably. This tub is made up of zinc. Three types of water temperatures are used for this bath. They are (1) Cold (2) Neutral and (3) Hot.

Method: The temperature of bath is maintained at 55°F-65°F by pouring cold water in the tub. The depth of the water is 2-2½ inches. The patient is asked to lie down inside the tub with the head on the elevated side and rest the legs on a small stool. Both hands can be kept on either side of the tub by the sides of the body inside the water. The duration of the bath can be from 10-20 minutes depending on the necessity.

In the absence of a spinal tub, a cold wet compress or a long rubber bag filled with cold water or ice can be applied to the entire spine. It will serve the same effect as that of cold spinal bath. After the spinal bath, the water should be wiped out immediately and the patient asked to bathe for 10-15 minutes. In case of weak patients, he is advised to lie on the bed covered with a blanket and bath to be taken after 30 minutes.

Physiological effects

Cold water is useful in reducing swelling and superficial congestion. It relaxes blood vessels and normalises blood circulation and body temperature.

Therapeutic effects

It is useful in relieving the congestion of brain, various types of vomiting, epilepsy, hysteria, insomnia, fever, constipation, sunstroke, etc. Cold spinal bath is also useful in extreme irritability of the body, e.g., burning sensation on the back in chronic eczema and psoriasis where there is no discharge. In **food** allergy, the symptoms of diarrhoea, vomiting, stomach-ache, etc. are controlled by cold spinal bath.

Contra-indications

In sciatica, paralysis, asthma, bronchitis, spondylitis, common cold, cough, backache and colics, such as uterine and renal colic, it is not applicable.

Hot/Neutral Spinal Bath

Method/Procedure: It is same as that of cold bath. The temperature of water is 105°F–115°F and 92°F–98°F respectively. Duration can vary between 15-60 minutes.

Therapeutic effects

It releases the nerve centres in the spinal cord, thus giving a calm and soothing effect on the viscera through the nerve filaments. It relieves nervous irritability and congestion of the brain, nervous system and cardiovascular system. It is very useful in cases of hypertension, insomnia and epilepsy. In case of **dust** allergy, the symptoms of sneezing, cold, cough, etc., are controlled by this method.

Spinal Spray

This is an important bath for treatment of diseases of the brain and spinal cord.

A spinal tub has been designed by Dr. Laxmana Sharma of Pudukottai, Tamil Nadu. This consists of a fibre glass tub with a perforated tube at the centre of the tub and a tank inside the tub having capacity of 40 litres. This tank is connected with a pipe to a 0.5 H.P. motor adjusted below the tub.

Ask the patient to lie down in the tub and start the machine. There will be a constant spray of ascending jet, which will give gentle massage to the whole spinal cord.

This is the most comfortable tub and also helps regulate temperature of water, i.e. cold, warm or neutral.

Therapeutic value of spinal spray

1. This procedure controls all the organs of the body, since most of the nerve roots start from the spinal cord. They are the sensory centres, temperature controlling centres, vasomotor centre and sympathetic and parasympathetic centres in the brain and spinal cord.

2. The hot or neutral spinal spray is useful for cases of **dust** allergy in which the small and large blood vessels of the lungs contract improving oxygen and blood supply to the lungs. It soothes the nerves and relieves the tension of the muscles and nerves after a day's hard work, and induces sound sleep at night.

3. The cold spinal spray is beneficial for cases of **food** allergy, wherein there is contraction of the digestive organs and their blood vessels, which relieves diarrhoea, vomiting and other gastric and intestinal disturbances.

Precautions

Very hot spinal spray can give rise to burns in the skin.

Heat Compress

A linen cloth or bandage of about 3 metres length and 30 centimetres width is kept in cold water for a few minutes. After squeezing it dry, it is bound around the abdomen in case of **food** allergy and chest and shoulder region in case of **dust** allergy. A dry woollen cloth or blanket is wrapped around it to prevent circulation of air and help accumulation of body heat. This has to be left in position for about an hour resulting in perspiration. After removing the compress, the area should be rubbed with a wet cloth and dried with a towel.

Hot Foot bath

This is the most useful and effective form of water treatment for many allergic disorders.

Procedure

A tub is filled with hot water in the temperature ranging from 102°F–122°F, depending on the tolerance of the individual. Alternately, the temperature may be gradually increased after every 2-3 minutes. The duration of the bath ranges from 10-20 minutes. Before starting the bath, the individual is asked to drink 1-2 glasses of water. A wet towel is kept on the head. After the bath, the feet must be kept in cold water for 1-2 minutes or rubbed with cold water using a towel followed by brisk drying with a thick towel.

Some naturopaths recommend a similar bath in which the hands and forearms are immersed in hot water up to the elbows. This should be done for 10 minutes twice or thrice daily.

Physiological effects

Hot foot bath dilates the blood vessels of the skin in the feet and draws blood from the congested parts of the body. By its reflex action it removes congestion from organs like the brain, lungs, digestive and genital organs.

Therapeutic effects

It is useful in **dust** allergy (sinusitis, asthma, bronchitis), **food** allergy, headaches of all types, insomnia, fatigue, mental tiredness, poor blood circulation, rheumatism, menstrual problems, renal colic, gout, neuralgia, etc.

Contra-indications

It is not applicable in high fever, hypertension, cardiac ailments, pregnancy, menstrual periods, prolonged fasting, fracture in legs, etc.

Friction Rub

The patient is made to sit at a tub with feet immersed in hot water up to the ankle. The face is washed with cold water. Some ice-cold water is taken in a basin and a coarse hand towel is dipped in the water. Each part of the body is rubbed briskly with this towel. After this, the body is covered with a bigger dry towel and rubbed again. This type of bath is very beneficial for patients with **food** allergy.

Alternate or Revulsive Bath

A tub is filled alternately with hot water between 105°F–115°F and cold water between 50°F–65°F. The patient should alternately sit in the hot tub for 5 minutes and in the cold tub for 3 minutes. The head and neck should be kept cold with a cold compress. The treatment should end with a spray of cold water to the body. This type of hydrotherapy is useful for both **dust** and **food** allergy.

Alternate hot and cold bath

This is done starting with a hot shower at 105°F for 4 minutes followed by a cold shower at 60°F for one minute. Repeat thrice, ending with a cold shower.

Mud Therapy

Earth provides us with food – our main source of energy. In the same way, earth, in the form of mud or clay packs or poultices or even mud baths, helps in the treatment and prevention of many diseases.

Mud therapy helps in activation of the metabolism by stimulating the endocrine and digestive organs. It also helps in the removal of impurities and toxins in the body.

How to Use the Mud

❏ Use commercially available mud or ordinary white clay. Spread it in the hot sunlight and allow it to dry. If it is very sticky, add some sand to make it fine. Sieve it well and remove stones, dirt and foreign particles. For best results, dissolve mud in water in a container overnight, filter it with a clean cloth and dry the filtrate.

❏ Always use mud with a clean stick or spatula and never with hands.

❏ In summer, mud should be dissolved in ice or cold water for better results and in winter it should be warm enough.

❏ For warm mud pack, boil water well and to it add mud.

❏ Mud, which is dissolved in water overnight, should be well covered to avoid contamination by dirt, dust, stones and impurities.

❑ Never re-use the mud which has been used for mud therapy.

Mud Therapy in the Treatment of Allergy

Mud Pack

❑ **For Food Allergy :** A thick cotton cloth soaked in cold water or ice with water squeezed out of it is applied on the abdomen. To this, apply a cold mud pack for 30 minutes. After removing the mud pack from the abdomen, apply a cold cloth. Repeat this procedure 3-4 times. In case of severe colicky pain in the abdomen, this procedure is done using lukewarm water.

❑ **For eye problems :** Apply wet clay pack on the eyes taking care to see that mud does not enter the eyes. This is a useful treatment for infections and inflammation of the eyes due to **dust** allergy.

❑ **For skin allergies :** Mud pack with multani mitti is to be applied on the affected area. After the mud dries, it should be washed with warm water, never with soap.

❑ **Allergy affecting the ears :** Fill the ear partly with cotton followed by wet clay. Apply warm mud pack outside the affected ear as well as around the neck and throat. This is useful for treatment of pain in the ear, boil inside the ear, discharge from the ear, etc. In acute cases, mud therapy should be preceded by fomentation of ear with cloth soaked in hot water. Mud pack is to be changed repeatedly.

❑ **Dust allergy :** A warm mud pack around the throat and neck and chest and upper back is very beneficial in controlling dust allergy affecting the nose throat and lungs (asthma).

❑ **For all allergies :** A whole body pack is prepared using a thick bedsheet and applying wet mud on it. The whole body is covered with the blanket in such a way that the mud spreads all over the body. Another bedsheet or blanket can be applied above the first bedsheet. Another way is to dig a pit up to the size of the patient. Cover with wet mud and make patient lie with head and neck uncovered.

Mud Bath

A mud bath may be taken using mud or earth from a place which has been exposed to direct sunlight and open air with no fertilisers used, and adequately hydrated. This mud or earth is mixed with some sand and water and applied to the whole body in the morning. The person should stay in the mild sunshine for about 30-40 minutes, applying mud whenever it dries up. At the end, a bath is taken with fresh water.

In some centres, a special tub is designed which allows people to lie in it covered up to the chin in mud. This allows them to lie comfortably in the tub for about 30 minutes, followed by a bath.

Massage

Massage is an excellent form of passive exercise as well as cure for many ailments. It is an integral part of Naturopathy as well as Ayurveda.

It tones up the nervous system activating each and every part of the brain. It accelerates the elimination of toxins and waste material from the body through the lungs, kidneys, bowels and skin. It also boosts up the blood circulation, digestion and metabolism.

Massage Useful for Treatment of Allergy

- ❏ Kneading
- ❏ Clapping
- ❏ Pounding
- ❏ Pressure vibration
- ❏ Stroking

Kneading

Kneading is a very important technique of massage used for treatment of allergy. Using both hands, deep pressure is exerted on the abdomen and lower back in case of **food** allergy and head, neck, chest and upper back in case of **dust** allergy. This is done for 10-15 minutes, preferably on an empty stomach in the morning.

This produces an increased flow of blood to the digestive and respiratory systems respectively, enhancing the process of digestion and respiration, absorption of nutrients, and removal of toxic products.

Clapping

This is a heavy movement used on the abdomen or chest, depending on the type of allergy. The patient is made to lie supine in such a way that the operator faces him from the right side. The upper abdomen is covered with a blanket. The operator (naturopath) strikes the abdomen with the inner aspect of right hand, with fingers loosely clenched and force transmitted from the shoulder.

The technique of clapping produces a mechanical stimulation of the abdomen/chest controlling their regular activities.

Pounding

This is similar to clapping except for the part that both the hands are used alternately on the abdomen/chest and the force used is slightly heavier.

This technique should be done only by an experienced naturopath.

Pressure vibration

Using one or both hands, vibrations are performed on the abdomen/chest. The movement is of fine shaking of the area by slight movements of the fingers or wrists. These movements have a soothing effect on the abdomen/chest, stimulating their activities.

Coarse vibrations can be done by keeping one hand on the back (spine) and the other on the abdomen/chest and moving the two hands with the breath held in expiration.

Stroking

For the treatment of allergy, slow and deep stroking of the abdomen/chest is recommended. It involves using finger tips of both hands slowly but with some pressure, and continuously in the concerned area. This movement relaxes the tightened and painful muscles and nerves, which in turn produces a soothing effect in these areas.

Medicated oils

For treatment of **food** allergy, massage may be done using almond oil, olive oil, mustard oil, sandalwood oil, coconut oil or pure "desi" ghee. These oils may be massaged on the abdomen and back preferably after warming, and on an empty stomach.

Medicated oils containing brahmi (Herpestis monniera), bala, amruta, ashwagandha, shatavari, gotu kola, bhringaraj and mandukparni have a cooling effect on the digestive system. Aromatic essential oils like lotus, peppermint, angelica, rose, mogra, lemon grass, khus, blue chamomile, clary sage, laudanum, rose gardenia, jasmine and lavender are also very useful in treating **food** allergy associated with vomiting and diarrhoea.

For **dust** allergy, massage with certain oils gives excellent results. The oils commonly used are cottonseed oil, sesame (til) oil, castor oil, mustard oil, olive oil and coconut oil. For better results, these oils are combined with eucalyptus, camphor, musk or myrrh.

Jojoba oil, along with essential oils such as cedar, pine musk, cinnamon, juniper, basil, ginger, cumin, cayenne, clove, yarrow, grapeseed, avocado and canola also give very good results in these patients. These oils are applied on the chest and back for 15-20 minutes, preferably on an empty stomach, followed by a warm water bath. For **skin** allergy, coconut and olive oils are very soothing.

12

Role of Ayurveda in Controlling Allergy

Treatment of allergy in Ayurveda is not just confined to medicines, diet and exercise but other measures are also involved. This difference in the approach to the disease is due to the difference in the concept of the disease. In Ayurveda, it is believed that any disease is due to imbalance in the doshas, i.e., one or more doshas may increase or decrease. Allergy is commonly believed to be due to increase in Vata dosha. In some individuals, depending on their inherent nature, there may be an increase in Pitta or Kapha doshas. Thus, the principle of treatment in Ayurveda is to bring about a balance in the three doshas.

For the sake of convenience, Ayurvedic treatment of allergy is divided into treatment of **dust** allergy, **food** allergy and **skin** allergy.

Ayurvedic Treatment of Dust Allergy

This is classified into two categories:-
- ❏ Treatment using Home Remedies
- ❏ Treatment using Classical Ayurvedic Medicines

Home Remedies

- ❏ Black tea prepared with black pepper powder, dry ginger powder and tulsi leaves. This tea can be taken

3-4 times a day to get relief from runny nose, headache and sore throat.

❏ Two grams of pure home-made turmeric powder well mixed in a cup of warm milk, taken twice a day effectively checks the cough. This should be continued for 15 days.

❏ 5ml of fresh tulsi juice well mixed in 10ml of pure honey, taken twice a day, calms down cough in children and adults.

❏ In chronic coughs, crush 1 or 2 garlic cloves, add to a glass of milk, boil the milk till ½ glass of milk remains, then filter it, add a little bit of sugar if desired, and divide it into two parts. Take one part in the morning and another in the evening. Do it for a week. There will be remarkable improvement. However, patients suffering from acidity should not use it, since it may aggravate the acidity.

❏ Similarly, onion juice can also be used. 5ml of fresh onion juice well mixed with 10ml of pure honey should be taken twice a day for 10 days.

❏ Steam inhalation of turmeric in water is very good for controlling cough.

❏ Take 1 teaspoon of besan (gram flour), roast it with 1 teaspoon of pure ghee. Add a cup of milk and 4-5 badams. Boil it for 2-3 minutes. It should be taken at bedtime. Water should not be taken after it.

❏ The juice of one clove of garlic (after removing the outer layer) is mixed with a tsp of honey and taken twice a day, to dilate the contracted bronchial tubes and dissolve mucus in the sinuses, bronchial tubes and lungs. Garlic foot bath is used by some French herbalists. A hot dish of garlic soup at bedtime is also soothing. Patients of ulcers and bleeding disorders should abstain from the above remedy.

❏ ½ tsp of hing (asafoetida), 50ml of sesame oil and a pinch of camphor are mixed and applied on the chest to relieve congestion and uneasiness.

- 1 tspful each of green ginger juice, betel leaf juice and juice of one clove of garlic are mixed and taken thrice a day, 1 tsp each time.

- Some camphor (karpur) and hing (asafoetida) are mixed well and pills of pea size are made. 1-2 pills taken with some hot water, 3-4 times a day, give relief.

- Pipal, amla and sonth taken in equal quantities crushed in the form of churana and taken with honey, mishri (sugar candy) and ghee give good results in mild attacks of asthma.

- Gur mixed with equal quantity of mustard oil taken for 21 days gives almost permanent relief from asthma.

- The powder of pipal taken along with sendha namak (rock salt) and mixed with the juice of ginger gives results in 7 days.

- Yoghurt inhibits production of histamine which produces symptoms of allergy. Goat milk yoghurt is best and should be preferably taken in the afternoon.

- Grape juice gives lot of energy, eliminates mucus and phlegm and cleans the blood toxins.

- Cranberries contain natural citric, malic and benzoic acids which act as intestinal antiseptics and facilitate digestion. They also contain a bronchial antispasmodic which dilates bronchial tubes. Cranberries may be cooked and mashed and taken with warm water or as juice.

- About 3-4 tablespoons of cooked asparagus may be taken twice daily or diluted with water to make a cold or hot drink.

- A cup of thyme (ajwain) tea with lemon and sugar helps in removing phlegm of the lungs in Bronchial Asthma. Herbal teas containing sage, comfrey, chamomile, eucalyptus leaves and garlic are useful in asthma.

❑ *Jushanda* is a popular remedy for Bronchitis. Take 1 teaspoon of this powder, add to it a cup of water. Boil it till half of it remains. Add some sugar or honey and take it at bedtime and in the morning before breakfast.

Classical Ayurvedic Medicines

❑ If amla is not available, its readymade preparation Amalaki rasayana in powder form is available in Ayurvedic stores. Take 3 grams of the powder along with warm milk twice a day.

❑ *Sitopaladi choorna*– a classical Ayurvedic preparation available in the stores, is a common drug. About 3-5 grams of this powder, mixed in 5ml of pure honey, should be taken twice or thrice a day. It works well for adults as well as children.

❑ *Lavangadi Vati* – one tablet thrice a day should be chewed. It controls throat irritation and cough rapidly. One can carry this while travelling.

❑ *Kaph-ketu Ras* – is another good preparation taken in the dose of 1-2 pills thrice daily with warm water.

❑ *Talisadi choorna,* 5gms + *Kapardika bhasma,* 1gm – should be given twice a day for 15 days.

❑ *Tribhuvan kirti Ras* – is the drug of choice for flu in the dose of 1-2 tablets crushed and mixed with honey taken 3-4 times daily.

❑ *Agastya rasayana* – is usually given to people who are asthmatics with constipation, sneezing, blocking of nostrils and congestion of throat.

❑ *Maha Laxmi Vilas Ras* – 1 tablet twice a day with *Triphala* quatha is a good remedy for sinusitis.

❑ *Chitraka hareetaki* – available in *lehya* form is a proven remedy. 2 teaspoons of this medicine should be mixed in a glass of warm milk, and taken twice a day.

❑ *Laxmi Vilas Ras* (Nardia) – 1 tablet thrice daily for the same period.

- *Shad Bindu Tail* – can be used for inhalation, 1 to 2 drops twice a day.

- *Talisadi churan* – taken ½ to 1 teaspoon along with honey and ginger juice gives relief in a day or two. The doses can be taken thrice a day.

- *Khadiravati* – should be kept in the mouth and sucked slowly. This gives relief in bronchitis associated with congested throat. 4-6 pills can be sucked over a day.

- *Vasarishta* – is a liquid taken 15ml in 15ml of water, twice a day after meals.

- *Haridara khand* – 5gm of it mixed with a cup of warm milk taken at bed time proves effective for **dust** allergy.

Ayurvedic Treatment of Food Allergy

Home Remedies

- A decoction of sandal (chandan) may be consumed thrice a day for relief from acidity due to food allergy.

- Tender fruit pulp of coconut may be taken from time to time. Tender coconut water soothes gastric irritation.

- About 200 to 500 ml of cold milk taken in sips during the day and at bedtime proves very beneficial in controlling acidity.

- Cardamom (elaichi) is a highly useful home remedy for gas. 5 grams of its powder can be taken with water. Take 5 grams each of fried asafoetida, commonly known as hing (by frying in ghee, hing becomes pure), black salt (commonly known as kalanamak), cardamoms (elaichi) and dry ginger known as sonth. Make a fine powder, mix well and store in a clean bottle. ½ teaspoon of this powder can be given along with some lukewarm water 2-3 times a day, which instantly gives relief from gas.

- Similarly, a mixture of 2 grams of ajmoda (celery seeds) and 1 gram saunph (aniseeds) and sugar (as required) is given in doses of ½ to 1 teaspoon with lukewarm water. This also gives prompt relief from gas problems.

- Take 1 part of hing, 2 parts of vacha, 3 parts of kala namak, 4 parts of sonth, 5 parts of jeera, 6 parts of harar, 7 parts of pohkar mul and 8 parts of kuth and prepare a choorna. Take about 3-5 gm of this choorna twice or thrice daily with warm water for immediate relief from gas.

- Amlaki – Botanically known as Emblica officinalis, Indian gooseberry is highly useful and the fresh juice extracted from the fruit along with some sugar, if consumed daily on empty stomach, works wonderfully in food allergy.

- Certain plants which have astringent properties like patol patar, brahmi, aloe, etc., are also very useful.

- The decoction of barley, pipal, parval along with honey can be taken for ulcers and acidity twice daily in the dose of 25 to 50ml.

- The powder of harar (2.5gm to 5gm) mixed with honey and gur has proved very effective for controlling food allergy.

- The decoction of dashmool taken in the quantity of 20ml mixed with 2.5gm powder of sonth taken twice daily gives immediate relief.

- The powder of harar and pipal taken in equal parts with warm water proves effective.

- Bel ki giri's powder, 2.5-5gm taken twice or thrice a day is very useful in controlling diarrhoea.

- The milk of goat boiled with equal quantity of water taken 20-50ml in divided doses gives relief in diarrhoea.

Classical Ayurvedic Medicines

❑ *Avipattikara choorna* – is a good Ayurvedic remedy. About 3 grams of powder, well dissolved in 50ml of hot water, should be taken twice a day for 40 days.

❑ *Sutshekar Ras* (simple) – 1 tablet thrice daily taken with water after meals controls acidity effectively.

❑ *Kamdudha Ras* (with pearls) – is a drug of choice for acidity taken in the dose of 1 tablet thrice daily.

❑ *Hingvastaka Choorna* – can be taken in a dose of 1 teaspoonful twice a day with hot water.

❑ *Hingutriguna Taila* – if given on empty stomach relieves constipation. The dose is 2 teaspoons once a day on empty stomach with a cup of hot water. This sets in bowel movement.

❑ *Kumar Asava* – an oral liquid, 20 ml with equal quantity of lukewarm water twice a day is also a good choice in gas problem.

❑ Besides these, *Leelavilas Ras, Chanderkala Ras, Amalpithantak Loh* are other useful medicines.

❑ *Kutaj Ghan Vati* – is very useful in diarrhoea. It should be taken as 1 tablet three times a day.

❑ *Sanjivini Vati* – is also commonly used by Ayurvedic physicians. It controls indigestion, flatulence and diarrhoea. The doses are 1 pill 2-3 times a day.

❑ *Kutajarishta* – 15ml mixed with equal quantity of water taken 2 times a day after meals can control diarrhoea due to **food** allergy.

Ayurvedic Treatment of Skin Allergy

Home Remedies

❑ The affected part should be cleaned daily with warm water boiled with the bark of the neem tree. This simple measure prevents secondary infections, and itching.

- The paste prepared from neem bark should be applied on the affected part and allowed to dry and then washed off.
- Pure neem oil, in a dosage of 2-4 drops well mixed in a cup of warm milk with sugar should be taken daily for 40 days.
- Doob grass, harar, sendha namak, chakbar and tulsi taken in equal quantities and crushed with kanji or buttermilk and applied on affected areas daily for 4-6 weeks gives good results.
- *Haridra* – is a popular home remedy. The powder should be taken as ½ tsp – twice daily with water.
- *Gairika* (red ochre) – is another popularly used remedy in this condition. One tsp of it, mixed with honey taken three times a day, is beneficial for skin allergy.

Classical Ayurvedic Medicines

Home Remedies

A number of effective, soothing ointment/oils are available which are to be used under the supervision of an Ayurvedic physician, since these contain arsenic, mercury, suphur, etc.

- *Pancha Tikta Ghrita Guggul* – A ghee-based pure herbal preparation – 2 teaspoonfuls well mixed in a cup of hot milk, should be taken on empty stomach, preferably in the early morning, followed by some warm water.
- *Khadirarista,* an oral liquid in doses of 20ml well mixed with equal quantity of water, should be taken twice a day after meals.
- For external application: *Guduchyadi Taila* – a medicated oil can be applied on the allergic patches as a primary drug.

- *Mahamarichayadi Taila* – is very effective for external application.
- *Panchnimbadi Churan* – ½ to 1 teaspoon twice daily taken with water after meals gives very good results in 15-20 days.
- *Sutsekhara Rasa* (simple) – 1 tablet three times a day.
- *Kamdudha Ras* – 1 tablet (of 125 mg) three times a day.
- *Haridra Khand* – 1 teaspoonful mixed with warm cup of milk at bedtime.

••

13

Homeopathic Treatment of Allergy

Homeopathy is derived from the Greek word "homeo" meaning like and "pathos" meaning suffering Homeopathy sees symptoms of disease as a positive outward sign that the body is trying to heal itself. Therefore, it holds that symptoms should not be suppressed as in the case of Allopathy and remedies are used which will help to stimulate and support the healing process.

A homeopath prescribes remedies for the "whole" individual, based on Hahnemann's three principles:-

❏ The law of similars

❏ The principle of minimum dose

❏ Whole-person prescribing

The Law of Similars

This law was formulated in 1796 and states that a substance that in large doses can produce symptoms of illness in a healthy person, can cure similar symptoms in a sick person if used in minute doses. Hahneman believed that this was because Nature allows for the existence of two similar diseases in the body at the same time. Homeopathic remedies work by introducing a similar artificial disease that negates the original disease, and yet its own effects are so minimal that it causes no suffering.

The Principle of Minimum Dose

This principle states that successive dilutions enhance the curative properties of a substance, while eradicating its side-effects. This means that the most minute dose of the substance is necessary for treatment of the disease.

Whole-person Prescribing

Homeopaths believe that the disease or its symptoms do not occur in isolation, but are an overall reflection of a person. Therefore, each person is treated as an individual based on his personality, temperament, emotional and physical state, likes and dislikes, before prescribing a treatment.

The Laws of Cure

Homeopathic treatment is believed to work according to a set of three rules or laws of cure. They are as follows:–

❏ A remedy starts healing from the top of the body and works downwards.

❏ It starts from within the body, working outwards and from major to minor organs.

❏ Symptoms clear up in reverse order to their manner of appearance.

Advantages of Homeopathy over other systems of Medicine

❏ It is the safest form of treatment with zero side-effects.

❏ It can be used by anyone – from babies, pregnant women to elderly people.

❏ While taking these medicines, alcoholic drinks, cigarettes, spicy or minty foods should be avoided.

❏ The medicines should be stored in a cool dark place in a tightly closed bottle away from strong perfumes, air fresheners or essential oils. If properly stored, the shelf life of these medicines is around 5 years.

❏ It is used worldwide with more than 100 million users in India.

- It is the only system of medicine which treats the patient as a whole taking into consideration his physical, mental and emotional factors.
- Treatment varies from individual to individual.
- It is painless and easy to administer.
- Invariably it is not expensive.
- There are no dietary or lifestyle modifications advised.
- It provides quick relief including cure in many cases.
- It does not suppress the symptoms but helps in boosting up the immune system for long-term results.
- Many surgical ailments and chronic diseases are cured with homeopathy.

How to use Homeopathic Remedies

- Take only one medicine at a time.
- Medicines should not be touched by hand, but transferred into the container lid or a clean spoon before transferring them into the mouth.
- Medicines should be taken after rinsing the mouth with water and preferably empty stomach or at least 30 minutes after meals.

Homeopathic Remedies for Allergy

For Dust Allergy, the medicines commonly used are as follows:-

- **Allergy affecting the eyes** – The useful remedies are Euphrasia (pills, and drops), Pulsatilla, Hepar sulfuris, Aconite, Mercurius solubilis (pus).
- **Allergy affecting the nose, throat and ear** – Kali bichromicum, Hepar sulfuris, Pulsatilla, Arsenicum album, Natrum muriaticum, Calcarea phosphorica, Sulfur, Allium, Gelsemium, Spongia.

❏ **Allergic Asthma** – The useful remedies are Arsenicum, Bryonia, Natrum sulfuricum, Lachesis, Ipecac, Antimonium tartaricum.

For Food Allergy, the useful Homeopathic remedies are:-

❏ **For nausea, vomiting, acidity** – the commonly used medicines are Sepia, Nux vomica, Arsenicum, Phosphorus, Pulsatilla, Arnica, Aconite, Anacardium, Kali bichromicum, Bryonia, China officinalis, Lycopodium, Graphites.

❏ **For abdominal pain, flatulence, diarrhoea** – the medicines are Lycopodium, Arsenicum, Argentum nitricum, Cantharis, Colchicum, Colocynthis, China, Phosphoric acid, Pulsatilla, Aconite, Mercurius, Sulfur, Baptisia.

For Skin Allergy

In Skin Allergy, the useful medicines are Urtica, Apis, Dulcamaera, Natrum muriaticum, Rhus toxicodendron, Sulfur, Arsenicum, Graphites, Aconite.

For Insect Bite Allergy

The immediate treatment of Insect Bite Allergy is to clean the affected area with pure tincture of Hypericum perforatum (St. John's Wort). Other useful medicines are Apis, Ledum, Arnica, Aconite (when associated with shock).

For Sun (Solar) Allergy

When associated with pain and burning sensation, Aloe vera, Allium hypericum (pills and ointment) Cantharis, Arnica, Urtica pills and ointment, Aconite are soothing and promote healing.

●●

14

Is Magnetotherapy the Solution to the Treatment

Magnetotherapy is a branch of medicine in which human diseases are treated by the application of magnets to the body of the patients. It is the simplest, cheapest and painless system of medicine with absolutely no side-effects.

Treatment of Allergy by Magnetotherapy

Dust Allergy

Dust allergy can be effectively controlled and even cured by using Magnetotherapy in the following ways:–

❏ The traditional treatment of allergy is to keep the North Pole of the high-power cast alloy magnet under the palm of the right hand and the South Pole under the palm of the left hand for 10 minutes twice daily. This helps in regulating the respiratory, circulatory and nervous systems.

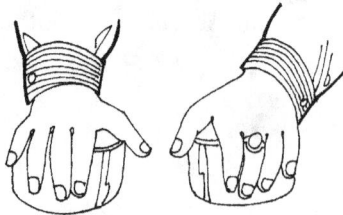

Fig. North Pole under right palm and South Pole under left palm

- North Pole of crescent (curved) type ceramic magnet should be applied on right nostril and South Pole on left nostril for 10 minutes twice daily. This will take care of nose-block, sneezing and watering from nose and eyes and ease the difficulty in breathing.

- If the same magnets are applied on the throat for 10 minutes twice daily, sore throat and dry cough can be reduced.

- Magnetic Necklace with 20 small magnets may be worn around the neck touching upper part of the chest. This may be worn throughout the day except when taking a bath. It can be also worn during the night.

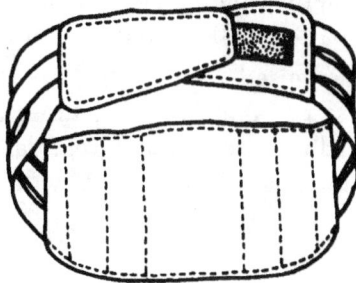

Fig. : Belly Belt

- Water magnetised with North and South Pole can be taken simultaneously in the dose of 50ml-75ml, 3-4 times daily for adults and in smaller doses for children, daily. This helps in removing congestion in the chest and lungs.

Food Allergy

- Keep the North Pole of the high-power cast alloy magnet under the palm of the right hand and the South Pole under the sole of the left foot for 10 minutes twice or thrice daily. This helps in regulating the digestive system and controlling symptoms of food allergy.

- Water magnetised with North and South Pole can be taken after every stool or vomitus in the dose of 50ml-75ml 3-4 times daily for adults and in smaller doses for children, daily.
- Specially designed belly (abdominal) belt can be useful for patients with food allergy. This belt is designed to cover the abdomen and back with magnets .This belt can be used for 30 to 60 minutes twice daily.

Insect Bite/Skin Allergy

- North Pole of the high-power cast alloy magnet should be applied directly to bitten or affected part immediately after the bite and for up to 10-15 minutes. For skin allergy, the magnet should be applied at the diseased part for 10-15 minutes thrice daily.
- Water magnetised with North Pole should be taken in the dose of 50ml-75ml, 3-4 times daily for adults and in smaller doses for children, daily. The affected part can be washed or dressed with the same water regularly.

Adverse Effects

These are very rarely seen, especially in those using high-power of electromagnets. The effects reported are as follows:

Mild tingling sensation in the hands and feet, a feeling of warmth in the body, heaviness of head, dryness of tongue, increased urge for urination, mild giddiness, and sweating in the areas on contact with magnets.

Precautions

- The ideal time for using Magnetotherapy is in the morning, preferably empty stomach and after a bath.
- Avoid eating or drinking cold things for at least one hour after applying high-power magnets.
- Since Magnetotherapy produces some heat in the body, bath should not be taken for at least one hour after treatment.

- If high-power or medium-power magnets are applied after full meals they may cause nausea.
- High-power magnets should not be applied to pregnant women, very weak ladies and to children.
- High power magnets should not be applied directly to delicate organs of the body, namely eyes, head and heart.
- Watches should not be allowed to come in contact with magnets unless they are anti-magnetic or magnet-proof.
- When high-power magnets are applied for long periods, they may produce heaviness in head, giddiness, yawning, tingling in nerves, etc. Discontinue contact with magnets and rest immediately.
- Opposite poles of high-power magnets should not be brought near each other face to face as they attract each other with great force.
- When high-power or medium-power magnets are not in use, they should be kept joined with a keeper so that their magnetism is not wasted and they are not demagnetised soon.
- When taking magnetic treatment under palms, it is not necessary to remove gold or silver rings from the finger.

●●

15

Benefits of Acupressure and Reflexology

It is believed that in our body there is presence of bioenergy or bioelectrical activity, which makes us move, breathe, eat and even, think. This energy is called "Prana" or "Chetana" in India while the Chinese call it "Chi" which consists of "Yin" or negative force and "Ÿang" or positive force. These forces or bioenergy flow through definite channels in the body called meridians or 'Jing'.

There are 14 meridians in our body of which 12 are located in pairs on either side of the body while the remaining two are single and lie each on the front and back of the body. The 12 paired meridians comprise 6 'Yin' meridians starting from the toes or mid-part of the body and reaching the head or fingers and 6 "Ÿang" meridians in the reverse direction.

These meridians maintain the flow of bioelectricity and are connected with the main organs or systems of the body. One end of each meridian lies in the hand, the leg or the face and the other in the main organ after which it is named. This is the reason why pressure applied to a particular point on the hand or the leg affects the remote organ connected with this point.

The 14 meridians are – large intestine meridian, stomach meridian, small intestine meridian, bladder meridian, triple warmer meridian, gall bladder meridian, lung meridian, spleen meridian, kidney meridian, heart meridian, heart constrictor or pericardium meridian, liver meridian, governing vessel meridian and conception vessel meridian.

Each of the 14 main meridians has subsidiary meridians. If the flow of bioenergy in a meridian is not proper, it can be corrected by stimulating certain points on the meridian by applying pressure on them. Thus the disease of that organ can be eliminated and the pain in these points is relieved as soon as the disease is eliminated.

Pain on any point on the body is possibly a symptom of some disorder in an organ or in a system of the body. If pressure is methodically applied on this point, the disease or disorder can be removed.

Effects of Acupressure

❏ It strengthens the body's natural resistance power due to which the functions of the lungs, heart and digestive system are normalised.

❏ In cases of allergy, the adverse effects of the allergens are minimised and even neutralised.

❏ Regular practice of Acupressure can sensitise the body to the unwanted and adverse effects of allergy and can almost cure a person of allergy.

❏ Acupressure can also normalise the respiratory rate, heartbeat, blood pressure, body temperature and metabolism of the body.

❏ There is also increase in the red and white blood cells and gamma globulins, and cholesterol and triglycerides are decreased.

❏ It reduces pain of different types, e.g., stomach-ache, joint pain, headache, backache, toothache, sprains, etc.

❏ It also has a tranquillising or sedative effect on the brain. If an EEG is done while doing acupressure, it shows depression of delta and theta waves.

❏ Depression, anxiety, stress and tension are controlled with acupressure due to its effect on the brain. This is also very beneficial for allergy.

❏ Muscles and joints are strengthened by Acupressure and are useful in the treatment of polio, paralysis and other neuromuscular disorders.

Advantages of Acupressure

❏ It is an easy, simple, effective form of treatment.

❏ It can be done in the privacy of one's home.

❏ Treatment can be done as frequently as possible.

❏ No money is required to be spent to get benefits of treatment.

❏ No side-effects are seen with this treatment.

❏ In this form of treatment, the person looks after his own health.

❏ In some cases, Acupressure can be used as a first aid measure till the doctor arrives or if the patient is admitted to the hospital.

❏ It helps prevent relapses of the diseases.

❏ If associated with other forms of treatment, it gives a speedy relief.

❏ It increases the efficiency of organs and systems of body, and strengthens joints and muscles.

❏ Even in serious diseases, it prevents aggravation of symptoms.

❏ It establishes the convention of touch communication or touch healing and establishes rapport between doctor and patient.

Reflexology or Zone Therapy

Reflexology refers to the form of treatment which involves giving massage to certain reflex areas of the feet and hands.

The body is divided into 10 longitudinal zones. If a straight line is drawn through the centre of the body, the whole body may be divided into five zones on either side of the body. Zone one extends from the thumb, up the arm to the brain and then down to the big toe, zone two extends from second finger, up the arm to the brain and down to the third toe.

Similarly, the other zones of equal width occur through the body from front to back. They are like segments of the body and not fine lines like acupuncture meridian lines. The line marking between each zone extends from the web of finger to the web of the toe. Whichever parts of the body are found within a certain zone, these parts will be linked to one another by energy flow within the zone and can therefore affect one another.

Treatment is done by applying pressure to accessible areas within the same zone. Pressure is applied using clothes pegs, metal combs, elastic bands and metal probes around the hands and fingers as well as toes, ankles, wrists, elbows or knees. The amount of pressure applied should be between 1kg and 9kg. for an interval of 30 seconds to 5 minutes.

The reflex areas of the feet and hands are divided into transverse zones. Zone one refers to all parts of the body above the shoulder girdle; Zone two refers to those parts between the shoulder girdle and waist; Zone three refers to organs below the waist.

Technique of Reflexology

The thumb is held bent and the side and end of the thumb is pressed into the part of the foot or hand to be treated. The other fingers of the hand will rest gently round the foot. Certain meridians are present in the sole of feet and their massage in the direction of flow of energy stimulates the organ. Massaging in the opposite direction gives a soothing effect.

Acupressure Points useful in the treatment of Allergy

Certain acupressure points and reflex centres when pressed are likely to result in reduction of allergic symptoms, as shown in these figures.

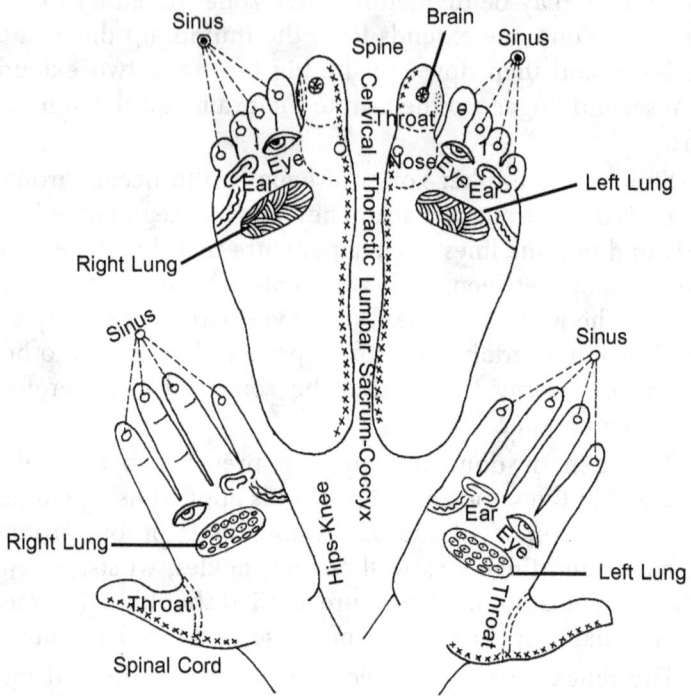

Fig. : Reflex Centres for Dust Allergy

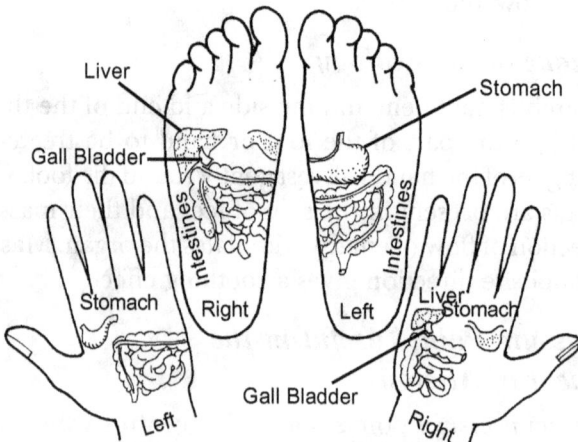

Fig. : Reflex Centres for Food Allergy

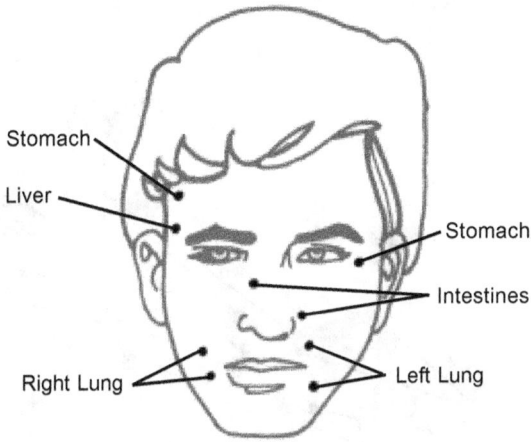

Fig. : Acupressure Points for Food Allergy

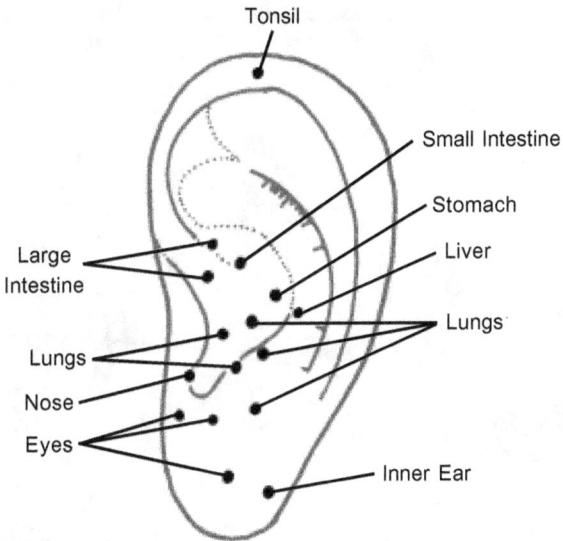

Fig. : Acupressure Points on the Ear

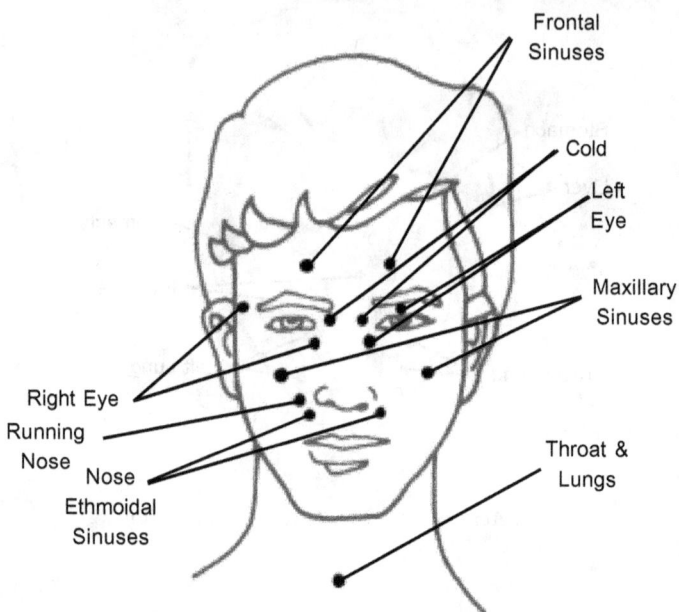

Fig. : Acupressure Points for Dust Allergy

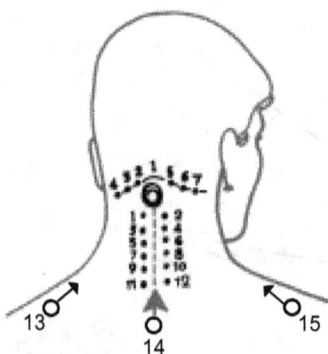

Fig. : Acupressure Points for Dust Allergy

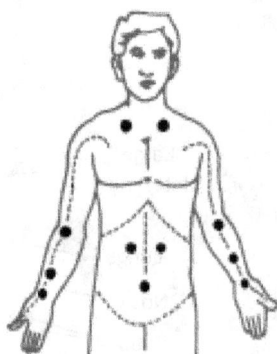

Fig. : Reflex Centres for Asthma

16

The Wonders of Colour Therapy (Chromotherapy)

Colour therapy or Chromotherapy refers to treatment of diseases using different colours. This is usually done in the following manner:–

- ❏ Direct radiation to the affected part/organ of the body.
- ❏ Application of oils, ghee, glycerine, etc., charged with specific colour to the affected part.
- ❏ Drinking water irradiated in specific coloured bottles.
- ❏ Using medicines charged with specific colours.
- ❏ Eating specific coloured food items.
- ❏ Inhaling gases charged in coloured containers.
- ❏ Wearing clothes of specific colours.
- ❏ Living/sleeping in a room painted with specific colours.

How it Works

Colour is a form of energy, which produces certain physiological changes in the body that help in controlling the disease and keeping the body fit.

According to colour therapists, every organ system has its own vibration energy and disease can occur when this energy is short. By applying these colours, the disease can be overcome. Modern Physics has established that every colour has a certain frequency wavelength and energy associated with it. Therefore the colour we absorb affects our neuroendocrine system and releases hormones and neurotransmitters which control the disease process.

Use of Colour Therapy in the Treatment of Allergy

Of the seven primary colours of the **Vibgyor** spectrum, certain colours are useful for the treatment of allergy depending on the type concerned.

For **food** allergy, **skin** allergy and **insect bite** allergy, the colours conventionally used are **Blue** and **Green,** while for **dust** allergy and **asthma,** the beneficial colours are **Orange** and **Red.**

The **red** and **orange** colours have a **stimulating** effect while the **green** and **blue** colours have a **soothing** effect and help in the repair of the disease process. Hence these colours are very beneficial for the treatment of allergy.

These colours act in the following ways:-

❏ They help in the stimulation of enzymes and chemicals, which overcome the adverse effects of different types of allergens.

❏ They increase the digestion of food substances including those, which may be allergic to the individuals by enhancing the function of digestive enzymes and annulling the toxic effects of these allergic food substances.

❏ They remove the toxins from the body and the blood.

❏ They activate the respiratory system helping in the expulsion of the aeroallergens, which lead to **dust** allergy and asthma.

❏ They activate the excretory systems like the urinary and lymphatic system, and enhance the process of excretion of toxins.

- ❏ These colours activate the mood and remove depression and help in overcoming stress.
- ❏ They control the blood sugar and prevent the deterioration in the function of pancreas, and also delay onset of complications.

Means of Applying Colour Therapy in the Treatment of Allergy

Direct Radiation

Take a little lamp and attach it with a green or blue coloured bulb or cover the existing bulb with green or blue coloured cellophane paper. Apply the direct rays of light from this lamp to the abdomen for about 10-15 minutes daily to overcome **food** allergy. The same procedure is applied for cases of **skin** allergy and **insect bite** allergy. In case of **dust** allergy and **asthma,** orange or red colours are applied on the chest, throat and back.

Local Application of Irradiated Oil, Ghee

Take a white or coloured bottle (depending on the type of allergy) and fill it with coconut oil, mustard oil, olive oil or ghee and place it on a dry wooden board exposed to direct sunlight for 45 days. It should be kept in the sunlight during the day and in a safe place at night. In case of cloudy/rainy days, artificial light may be used.

This irradiated oil can be used to massage the abdomen, chest, throat or affected skin region.

Drinking Irradiated Water

Using the procedure given above, water can be charged in the required coloured bottles. This should be drunk in the dose of 1 cup early in the morning and ½ cup before lunch and dinner. This will help in eliminating the allergens from the body

Inhaling Coloured "Air"

An empty red or orange coloured bottle is kept in the sunlight for about an hour. After removing the cork, the sun-charged "air" in the bottle should be inhaled for a few minutes. This should be repeated thrice daily. This therapy can improve the function of the respiratory system and help in the treatment of **dust** allergy.

Eating Specific Coloured Food Items

Consuming fruits and vegetables, which are red or orange in colour, can also help in the treatment of **dust** allergy. Examples of such fruits and vegetables are carrots, oranges, apples, apricots, peaches, red berries, water-melon, beet root, radish, red cabbage and red spinach.

Since blue and green colours soothe the mind and body, consuming fruits and vegetables of such colours can be useful in cases of **food** and **skin** allergy.The fruits and vegetables of such colours are blue plums, blue berries, black berries, blue grapes, purple grapes, phalsa, jamun, egg plant, purple broccoli, beet tops, black carrots, kanji of black carrots, viola odorata (banafsha) and several green leafy vegetables and fruits.

Clothing

Wearing blue or green coloured clothes can prove to be very useful for people with **food** allergy while red, orange and even yellow can help individuals with **dust** allergy. Wearing night-suits and sleeping on a bed with bedsheet, pillows and bedcovers of the above colours can give rise to reduction in above allergies. In case of asthmatic attacks, tying of a 4-inch wide cotton scarlet red colour bandage on the left forearm at the wrist or above has shown spectacular results.

Colour Scheme in the Bedroom

If the bedroom walls are painted with above colour schemes and the furniture and other items are of the same colour in the bedroom, it can create wonders. If such individuals wear similar night-dress and have the same colour combination with bedding, lighting, etc., there can be no problem in controlling allergies.

●●

17

Can Music Therapy be of Some Benefit

Music Therapy is a form of treatment using music and musical instruments in order to restore, maintain and improve physical, physiological, psychological and spiritual health and well-being.

Benefits of Music Therapy

Music therapy, when used, brings about following benefits or changes in patients and individuals:–

- ❏ It produces reduction in anxiety and stress, often producing sedation and even sleep.
- ❏ It can alleviate pain and discomfort in conjunction with anaesthesia or pain medication.
- ❏ It can bring about positive changes in mood and emotional states.
- ❏ It can counteract apprehension or fear.
- ❏ It can lessen muscle tension bringing about relaxation of the body.
- ❏ Music therapy brings about active participation of the patient in his treatment.
- ❏ The length of stay in the hospital or treatment period is decreased.

❏ An emotional bond develops between the patient, his family members and the doctors.

❏ This type of therapy is enjoyed by all.

❏ The whole period of therapy forms a meaningful time spent together in a positive and creative way.

❏ It improves communication skills and physical coordination in spastic and mentally retarded patients.

Medical Application of Music Therapy

Music therapy has been found to be useful in the treatment of the following diseases:-

Sleep disorders, behavioural disorders in children, mental retardation, stammering and speech disorders, psychiatric illnesses like anxiety neurosis, depression, schizophrenia, dementia and Alzheimer's disease, arthritis, stroke, acute and chronic pain, hypertension, polio, tinnitus, epilepsy, polio, drug addiction and head injury.

How Music Therapy Helps Patients of Allergy

❏ It increases the digestive and metabolic activity in the body – increasing the secretions of digestive enzymes and hormones. This can lead to counteracting the adverse effects of food allergens in case of **food** allergy.

❏ The immune system is boosted up which helps in combating various types of allergies which are mainly due to abnormality in the immune system.

❏ Music Therapy improves the breathing activities in the body and helps in expelling or reducing the adverse effects of aeroallergens.

❏ Mental stress and tension, which is a major factor in allergy, is controlled by reducing the levels of stress hormones in the body.

❏ It stabilises the blood pressure and heart rate and hence prevents complications of the heart. There is improvement in the cardiac output or blood circulation, which invigorates the whole body.

- ❏ Active participation in music and dance enhances activity of nerves and muscles and prevents onset of neuromuscular complications.
- ❏ There is a vast improvement in mood and behaviour of the individual.
- ❏ There is an increased sense of well-being and optimistic approach to life.

The Ragas Useful for Treatment of Allergy

Research done in the medical application of Music has shown that the following Ragas are useful in the treatment of allergy:

Raga Kalingara, Raga Hindol, Raga Bhairav, Raga Kafi, Raga Hansdhwani, Raga Bihag, Raga Malkauns, Raga Ramkali, Raga Bahar, Raga Deshkar, Raga Lalit, and Raga Jaijaiwanti.

●●

18

The Role of Vastu Shastra and Feng Shui

Vastu Shastra and Feng Shui

Vastu Shastra refers to the age-old Indian tradition of undertaking auspicious events and tasks based on the basic directions – North, South, East and West or while constructing a house. Feng Shui is the ancient Chinese art of living in harmony with the environment. It uses "chi" (energy) to determine the positive and negative aspects of a home, office, building or factory environment.

Basic Philosophy

Vastu Shastra is based on the basic concepts of the sun's energy, which is maximum in the East and certain auspicious areas/directions related to Brahma, Vishnu and Shiva. Feng Shui is based on the theory that there is an invisible energy that flows through the universe, through our body, the food we eat, our home and workplace and the environment around us. It is known as "prana" in India; "Chi" in China and "ki" in Japan.

According to a map or "Bagua", living space is divided into nine areas – career, knowledge, health, wealth, fame, relationships, children, travel and good luck. Energising of these respective areas can enhance these qualities or areas of life.

	South		
East	Wealth	Fame	Relationship	West
	Health	Good Luck	Children
	Knowledge	Career	Travel
	North

How it works

It mainly works through colour schemes, placement of furniture, lighting, plants and reflective objects such as sculptures, paintings and art. To produce proper impact, they should be so arranged that they are harmonious with the forces of Nature or cosmic energy. Hence, one can improve one's health, wealth, relationship, knowledge, career, etc.

Vastu and Feng Shui Measures for Treatment of Allergy

The **Health sector** or the **eastern portion of the house** should be organised in such a way that all people, especially those suffering from allergy can live a long and healthy life. These measures are as follows:

❏ This room should be well-illuminated to allow increased amount of light, which enables increased flow of "chi" into this part of the house.

❏ Potted plants encourage good health and should form an integral part of the room.

❏ Photographs of family members and objects given by relatives, friends and well-wishers should be kept in the health sector.

❏ An aquarium or pictures depicting rivers, streams, waterfalls or lakes help in the well-being of occupants of the house.

❏ Keeping metallic wind chimes with hollow rods at the entrance or in the eastern portion help in the flow of beneficial "chi" and remove all negative influences, especially bad health.

117

- Keeping an orange or yellow coloured bulb or candle lighted in this room during night is also useful.
- Painting the walls of the room with orange or yellow paint can keep all the occupants of the house fit and fine.
- There should be no clutter or useless things in this room, which impede the free flow of energy into this room.
- The atmosphere can be further energised in this room by regular burning of incense or performing havan or kirtan regularly.

Measures pertaining to the bedroom and other areas of the house

- The bedroom should be ideally located in the South-west portion of the house known as the sector for marriage and romantic happiness.
- If it is not possible to allocate the bedroom in this sector, the bed should be so aligned that the head points preferably towards the South-west or South. This allows the "chi" energy to flow into the body while sleeping.
- The head or the feet should not point towards the door while sleeping since these are known as "coffin positions."
- If there is an attached toilet or bathroom in the bedroom, the occupants should not face the entrance to this room because they will breathe in negative "chi" throughout the night.
- If the long side of the bed is against the same wall as the entrance, one should not sleep with his back to the wall.
- The bed should not be lying under an exposed beam on the ceiling. In case there is no alternative, the bed should be placed in such a way that the beam runs parallel to the bed and not across it. As a remedy,

118

two bamboo flutes can be hung from the beam, tied with red thread or ribbon.

❏ The bedroom should receive sufficient light during the forenoon while the curtains may be drawn in the afternoon and night.

❏ The dressing table should face South-west but never the foot end of the bed.

❏ Never keep anything related to the office or do office-work in the bedroom.

❏ Keep metallic wind chimes with hollow rods in the bedroom, which help in the flow of beneficial "chi" flowing through the home whenever they move. Alternately, hanging a crystal can provide positive energy and avoid nightmares.

❏ Coloured lights based on the beneficial colours mentioned in the chapter on Colour Therapy and painting of the bedroom walls create a relaxed atmosphere in the room and prevent unnecessary health problems while in the bedroom. Burning a small blue or violet candle in the bedroom every evening is also useful.

❏ All electrical appliances in the bedroom should be unplugged or switched off at night or persons should sleep at least 4 feet away from these appliances. This is to avoid man-made electromagnetic fields or radiations.

❏ Keeping hibiscus in the bedroom promotes sexual compatibility and is a stress-buster. Jasmine is considered to be an aphrodisiac and anti-depressant. Tulsi plant helps in keeping away evil thoughts and arresting the negative energy of any visitor entering into the house.

❏ The bathroom and toilet should not be in the northern side of the house. If present, avoid using it or keep the lid down and door closed. A large mirror may also be placed outside its door to symbolically make it disappear.

●●